We dedicate the two books we have written on how to incorporate isometric exercises into golf to improve strength, agility, and overall performance to Simon Earle.

Simon, a cancer survivor, has not only been a lifelong golfer but also a close friend to both authors. His journey, marked by resilience and a positive attitude, is a testament to his strength and character.

Simon's recovery journey was not just about surviving cancer but about thriving. He used a combination of regular isometric exercise and golf, not just as physical activities but as powerful tools to maintain his trademark positive mental attitude. His story is a beacon of hope and inspiration for all.

Isometric Exercises for Golf™

Part 1. Exercises for Individuals

Strength, Muscle and Stamina Building Exercises to Improve Your Game and to Perform During Your Game

Published by

MajorVision International

2020

△ | TWiEA
The World Isometric Exercise Association

Approved by The World Isometric Exercise Association
www.TWiEA.com

Copyright and Trademark Notice
© 2020 Brian Sterling-Vete and Helen Renée Wuorio
All Rights Reserved

All material in this book is the property of, copyrighted, and trademarked to Brian Sterling-Vete and Helen Renée Wuorio and/or MajorVision Ltd; unless otherwise stated, A E & O E. Copyright and other intellectual property laws protect these materials. Reproduction, distribution, or transmission of the materials, in whole or in part, in any manner, without the prior written consent of the copyright holder is prohibited and is a violation of national and international copyright law.

www.HelenRenee.com – www.BrianSterlingVete.com

Contents

Important General Safety and Health Guidelines
Introductory Notes and Precautions
- Special Precautions When Using Golf Clubs as Exercise Tools

1. **Golf – The Great Game**
   - Golf as Exercise
   - What Muscles are Engaged During a Golf Swing?
   - A Golfer's Walk is a Healthy Walk
   - Golf Clubs - Overview
   - Golfer's Elbow

2. **Exercise Science Overview**
   - Walking Vs Running as a Fat Burner
   - Walking, General Activity and N.E.A.T. - Non-Exercise Activity Thermogenesis
   - The Basic Types of Resistance Exercise
   - Isometrics
   - Isometric Exercise Science
   - The Standard Isometric Contraction
   - Intensity, Force, Strength, and Power
   - Technically, How Does a Muscle Grow?
   - Rest and Recovery
   - Rest Time Between Exercises
   - Dynamic Flexation™
   - Isometric Exercises and Blood Pressure

3. **Proprietary Isometric Exercise Equipment**
   - Securing the Iso-Bow® With Your Feet

4. **About the Exercise Model**
5. **Things to Remember Before You Begin**
6. **Exercise Resources**
7. **Conclusion**
   - What is TWiEA™?

www.HelenRenee.com – www.BrianSterlingVete.com

Important General Safety and Health Guidelines

The contents of this book are strictly the experiences and opinions of the authors and are not intended to serve as a guide or instruction manual for exercise.

The authors are not medical professionals, and the information presented should not be construed as medical advice.

It is imperative that the reader consult with a qualified healthcare provider before implementing any exercise routines, techniques, or implied recommendations in this book.

The reader should not undertake any exercise regimen without obtaining the full approval of their physician.

The authors and publisher assume no liability for any injuries, damages, or adverse effects that may result from the use of the information provided in this book.

It is the reader's responsibility to ensure that any exercise programme or changes to their physical activity are appropriate for their individual health status and are undertaken under the supervision and guidance of their medical doctor.

Use and Copyright:

The contents of this book are protected by copyright laws. Participants are prohibited from reproducing, distributing, or sharing the coursebook or its contents without the written consent of the creators.

The creators and instructors of this book are not responsible for any unauthorised use, reproduction, or misuse of the book's contents.

Conclusion:

By reading this book, you acknowledge and accept the limitations of liability of the creators and authors and agree to adhere to the provided guidelines and safety precautions.

It is essential to consult with healthcare professionals before undertaking any physical exercise activity.

For additional general information, we also recommend that you check reputable accredited medical advice sites, such as:

The National Health Service in the United Kingdom, online at:

https://www.nhs.uk/Livewell/fitness/pages/physical-activity-guidelines-for-adults.aspx

And/or The Mayo Clinic in the USA:

https://www.mayoclinic.org/healthy-lifestyle

Introductory Notes and Precautions

This book is one of two companion books called Isometric Exercises for Golf™. Part 1 focuses on different exercises from those in Part 2. However, both books detail the overall benefits of isometric exercise and how to perform it to enhance the golfing experience. These exercises can be performed during a game, during breaks in practice, at home in your lounge, or anywhere else you choose.

The first book (Part 1) is entirely dedicated to exercises that can be performed individually, and the second book (Part 2) is entirely dedicated to exercises that can be performed in pairs with an exercise buddy.

The technical introductions in both books will contain either the same or virtually the same information. This is because the underlying exercise science of isometric exercises does not change, nor does the science about how muscle grows, and how fat is burned, etc.

Both books contain detailed information describing how to perform exercises that target, strengthen, and tone all the main parts of the body. They also contain large descriptive pictures together with arrows that indicate the suggested direction in which the exercise force should be applied.

The exercises are not laid out in a course format. Instead, they are listed to show what exercises can be performed for each body part so that individuals and fitness professionals can simply choose which to perform according to their objectives.

Since both books contain all the essential information for exercising either individually or with an exercise buddy, if someone chooses to read only one of them, they will be fully prepared.

This means that, depending upon the objective, either or both books can be used as valuable stand-alone resources in the field by professional golf coaches who wish to help their clients improve their strength and fitness and their golf game.

This shared introduction process for this topic also means that if someone already owns one book, they have already read the critical information about the exercise system and can go directly to the exercise section if they decide to buy the other. However, we would always recommend that everyone recaps the important health, safety, and health guidelines every time.

Perhaps the most important benefit is that if the isometric exercises are practised regularly at home, either as an individual or with a partner, they will greatly improve one's overall strength, fitness, and endurance for golf and life in general.

The exercises listed in this book, Part 1., are designed to be performed alone, without the need for an exercise partner, so they will need to be adapted to be practised with a partner. Some exercises may not directly interchange, so you must find alternative exercises for the same body part/muscle group.

Therefore, we suggest that if you wish to exercise with a partner using the highly effective isometric system, you get a copy of Part 2 and/or The ISOmetric Bible™ (also available on Amazon), which is one of the most comprehensive and detailed isometric exercise books available today.

At the end of this book is a list of other books about fitness, healthy living, well-being, muscle, and strength building.

Special Precautions When Using Golf Clubs as Exercise Tools

Remember that when using golf clubs as exercise tools, one should always be extra cautious. Clubs may inadvertently slip out of your hand/s at any time without notice, so be sure to take this into consideration and exercise with enough safety distance between you and anyone standing next to or generally near you.

Golf clubs may slip on the ground without notice, so always be aware of this possibility and take precautions in advance, just in case.

Golf clubs with any kind of adjustable joints or handle, etc., may fail at any time without notice, and no matter how unlikely this may be, one should always be aware of this possibility and be prepared for it.

If in any doubt about the structural integrity of any kind of golf club or improvised isometric exercise tool, then do not use it for exercise or any other purpose.

Chapter 1: Golf – The Great Game

In its most basic form, golf is a club-and-ball sport where players use various types of clubs to hit golf balls into a series of holes on a course in as few strokes as possible. It sounds easy, doesn't it? However. It is highly addictive, lots of fun and often extremely frustrating.

The modern game as we know it today originated in 15th-century Scotland, with the first written record of golf being when it was banned by James II in 1457 because it was seen as an unwelcome distraction to learning archery. Thankfully, James IV lifted the ban in 1502 when he became enticed over to the *dark side* and a golfer himself! Beyond these recorded beginnings, the game's ancient origins remain unclear and are often debated.

Some historians have traced golf back to the Roman game of paganica, in which participants used a bent stick to hit a stuffed leather ball. It is surmised by some that paganica then organically spread throughout Europe as the Roman Empire spread across the continent during the first century BC and that paganica eventually evolved into the modern game. Other ancient games that resemble modern golf and could at least in part have contributed to the modern game were known as cambuca in England and chambot in France; the Persian game, chaugán, is another possible ancient origin, and kolven, which was played annually in Loenen, in the Netherlands from around 1297 onwards.

Golf was first 'exported' to the United States by two Scotsmen from Dunfermline. Robert Lockhart and John Reid first demonstrated golf in the U.S.A. when they set up a hole in an orchard in 1888. Later the same year, John Reid set up America's first golf club, which quite naturally was called Saint Andrew's Golf Club in Yonkers, New York, paying homage to the 18-hole round course created at the Old Course at St Andrews, Scotland, in 1764. The rest, as the saying goes, is history.

Additional exercises can be performed during break times enjoyed by most recreational golfers to greatly increase golf's health, fitness and strength-building benefits. Interestingly, an increasing number of golf professionals are now allocating time for specific improvised exercise sessions during golf coaching sessions with clients.

Perhaps the easiest and most effective form of exercise to engage in during a walking break is isometric. This is because it can be safely performed by almost anyone of any age, requires no special equipment, and still delivers optimum results.

Also, it can easily be performed and enhanced by incorporating the use of golf clubs as simple but highly effective isometric exercise tools.

What is it about a golf club that makes it a good IIED or Improvised Isometric Exercise Devices? The golf club, by its very size, weight, and the material from which it is constructed, make it an ideal portable isometric exercise tool. The shaft of a golf club is typically a strong tapered metal tube, usually steel) or carbon fibre composite, AKA graphite. The shaft is typically approximately 0.5 inches (13 mm) in diameter near the grip and between 34 to 48 inches (86 to 122 cm) in length. A typical shaft weighs between 45 to 150 grams (1.6 to 5.3 oz), depending on the material and length.

Why isometric exercise and not traditional isotonic callisthenics? It is never an either-or scenario because the type of exercise an individual prefers is entirely their own business. Both isotonic and isometric exercises deliver excellent results; however, it is also just a fact that isotonic exercises typically take longer to perform and require more space and movement than isometric exercises. Also, the optimum time an isometric exercise should be performed is 7 seconds. This means that if you perform one simple isometric exercise at each of the 18 holes on a golf course, then you will have performed a comprehensive total-body isometric exercise workout at the end of a typical game of golf. You will have strengthened and toned all the major muscles without breaking a sweat or your concentration from the game of golf itself.

It should also be noted that isometric exercise is one of the most well-researched exercise techniques and has been proven to be superior to many other types of exercise in terms of delivering maximum results for minimum effort in terms of muscle, fitness and general strength-building. Therefore, this is the exercise technique we will focus on.

A growing number of professional golf coaches are also qualified and certified to teach clients isometric exercises that can be used during practice sessions, breaks during golf, or at home.

More information about these instructors and how to find them can be found at TWiEA.com, where some approved isometric exercise instructors are listed together with information about how golf and other fitness professionals can become qualified to teach isometric exercise to enhance the overall golfing experience for their clients.

Golf as Exercise

Some view golf as an excellent form of exercise combined with a frustratingly addictive, fun-filled game, while others view it as something that spoils a nice walk. Golf is always going to be perceived differently depending on whether you are a fan or not.

However, for those people who view golf as something that spoils a nice walk, there are some particularly important points to consider. Playing golf does much more than provide a good reason to walk outdoors for several hours. The complex physical actions involved in playing the game exercise a lot of muscles in the process; in fact, many more than one might at first think.

What Muscles Are Engaged During a Golf Swing?

Perhaps the most obvious muscles used are those of the forearm because unless you grip the club, you simply cannot play the game, let alone send the ball flying in the right direction. The hand, wrist, forearm, triceps, and biceps muscles are all essential to developing a powerful golfer's swing.

Making all these muscles stronger will, without question, improve your overall game. The main forearm muscles engaged during a golf swing are the flexors, the flexor digitorum profundus, the flexor pollicis longus, to a degree, the extensors, and the digiorum superficialis.

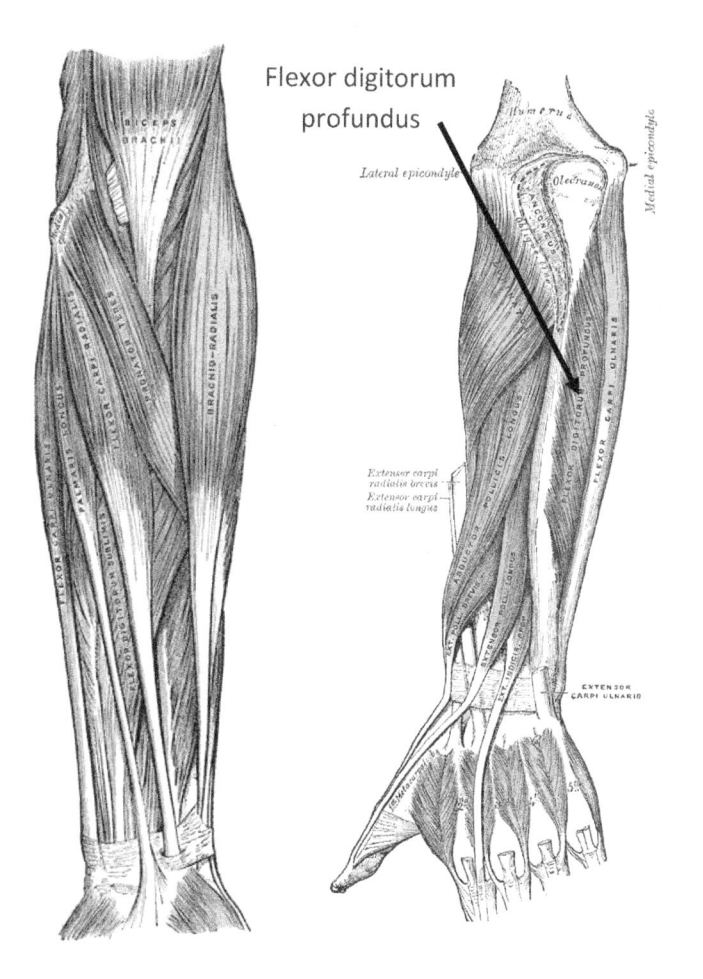

Flexor digitorum profundus

The biceps and triceps muscles of the upper arm are essential to a good golf swing. Therefore, both sexes should exercise to tone and strengthen them. In addition, these muscles help give the arms an athletic and toned appearance, so exercising them will help your appearance aesthetically, too.

Biceps

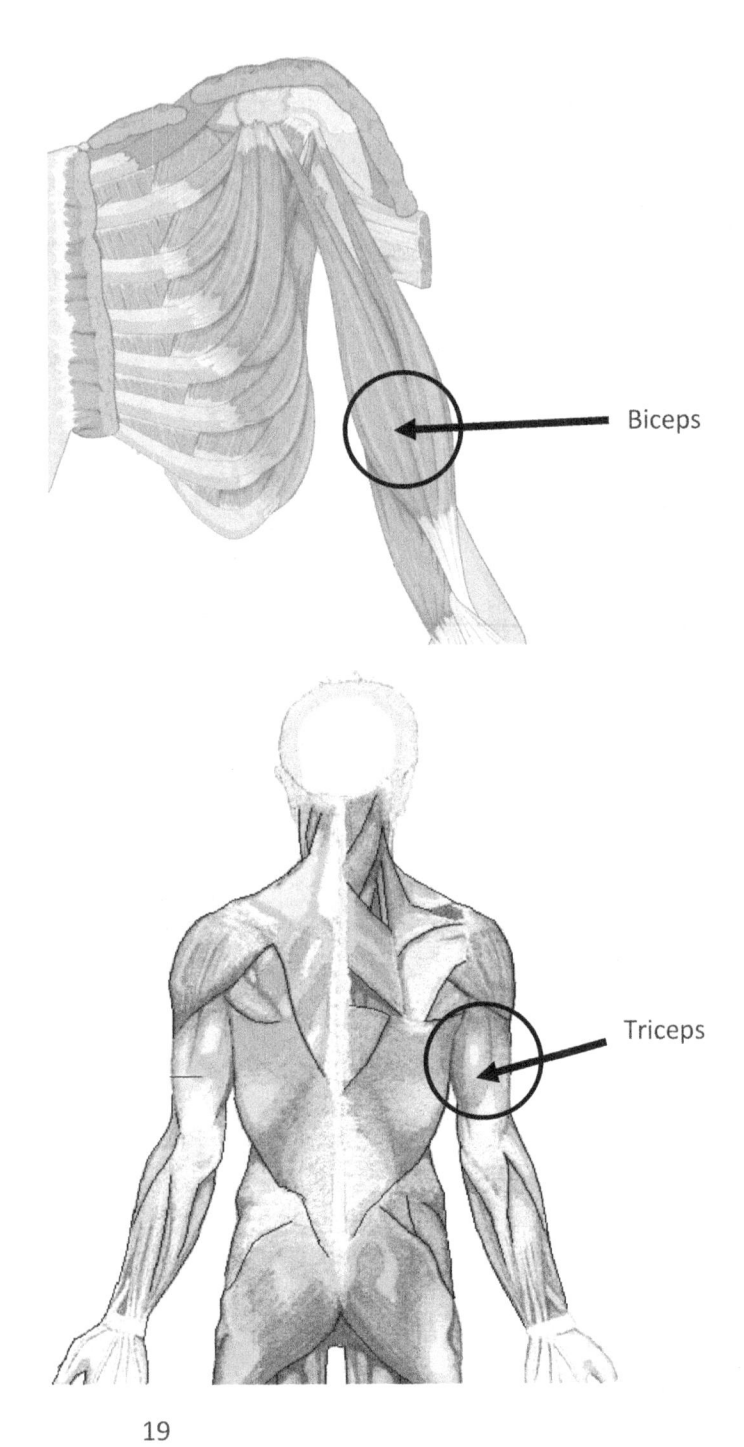

Triceps

Strong core muscles are the basis of a good golf swing, and strong and flexible core muscles will stabilise your entire body and support your spine. In particular, the abdominal external oblique muscles are engaged when rotating the torso and are located along the side of the torso and the sides of the ribs from under the arm to the crest of the hip. Other muscles involved are the multifidus, the rotatores, and the erector spinae.

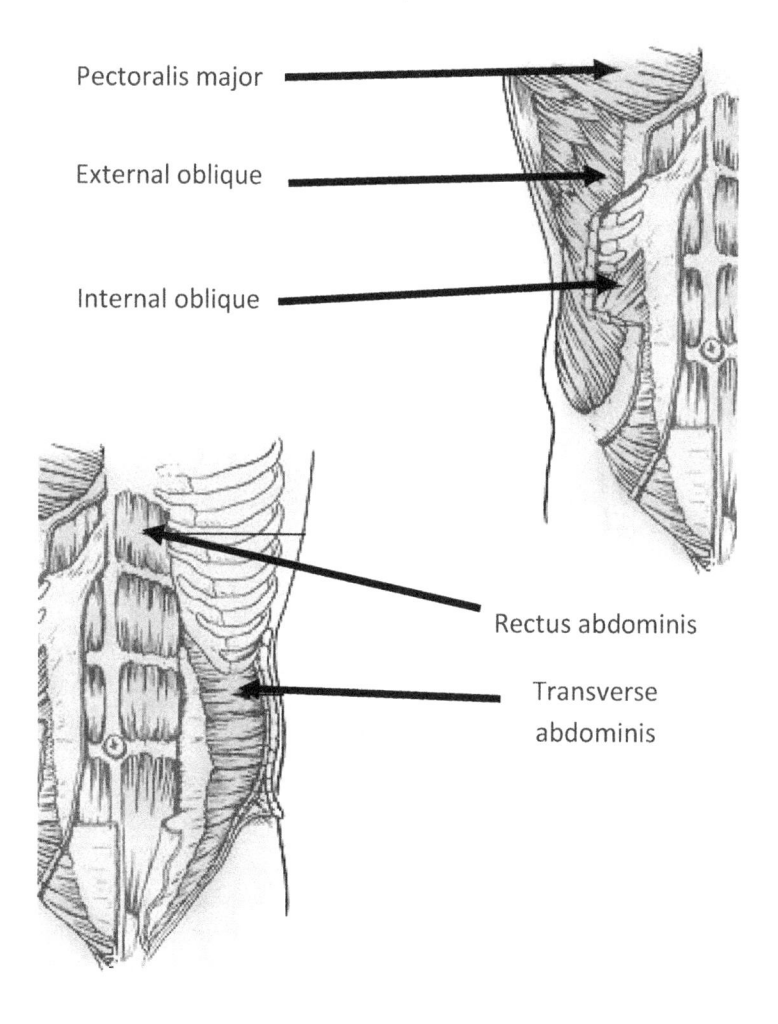

Pectoralis major

External oblique

Internal oblique

Rectus abdominis

Transverse abdominis

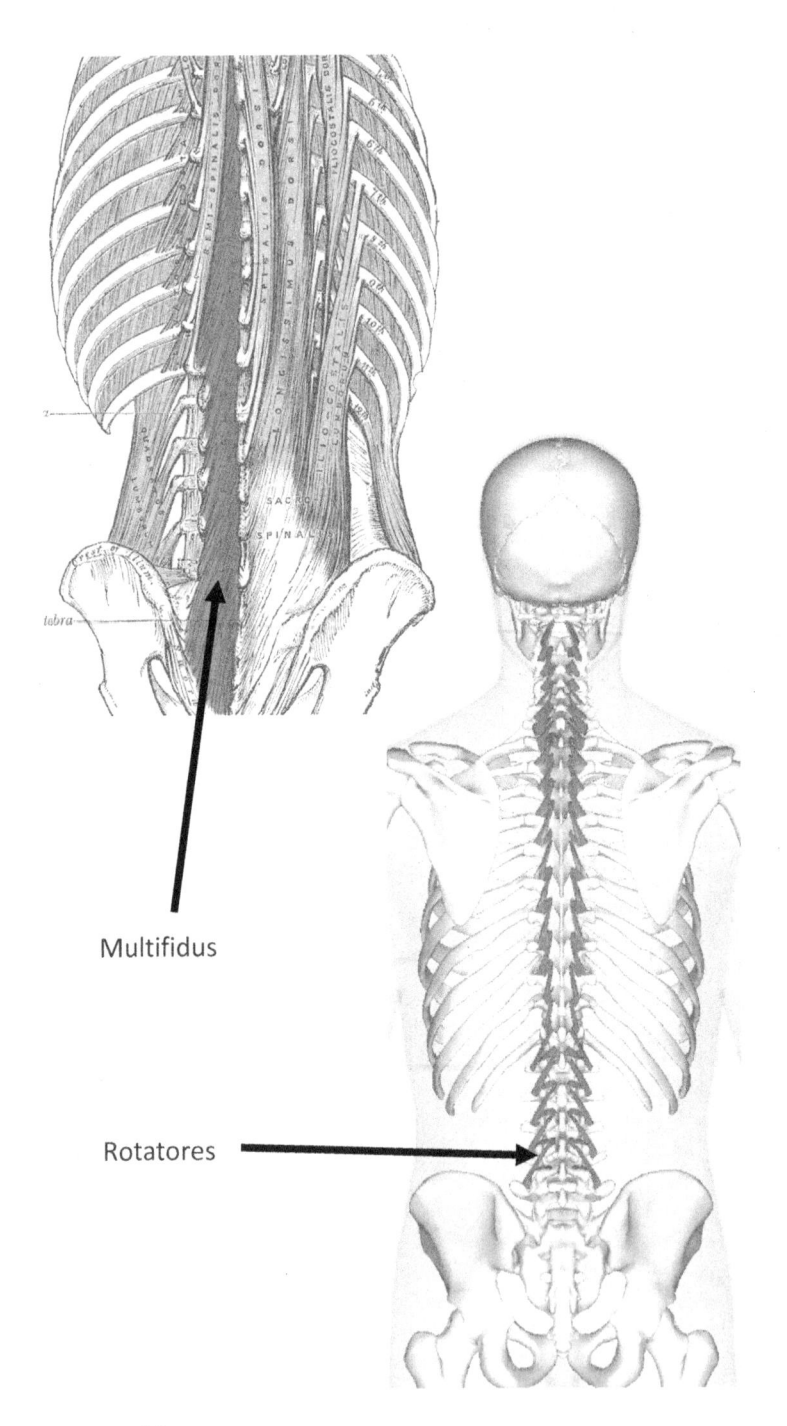

Multifidus

Rotatores

The muscles of the upper back control the backswing and follow-through with the golf club. The primary upper back muscles engaged during a golf swing are the latissimus dorsi. The latissimus dorsi give the classic 'V' shape to the torso and are located extending from underneath the arm to the mid-level of the back. The latissimus dorsi connects to the shoulder blade (scapula) and the ribs in the thoracic area. The latissimus dorsi enable the golf swing to move towards the body (adduct), then help rotate the body and extend the body through the outward swing. Any lack of flexibility in the upper back muscles can lead to a shorter, irregular swing and limited follow-through. Therefore, as well as performing strengthening exercises it is also important to perform proper stretching as this will help to develop a longer, faster swing.

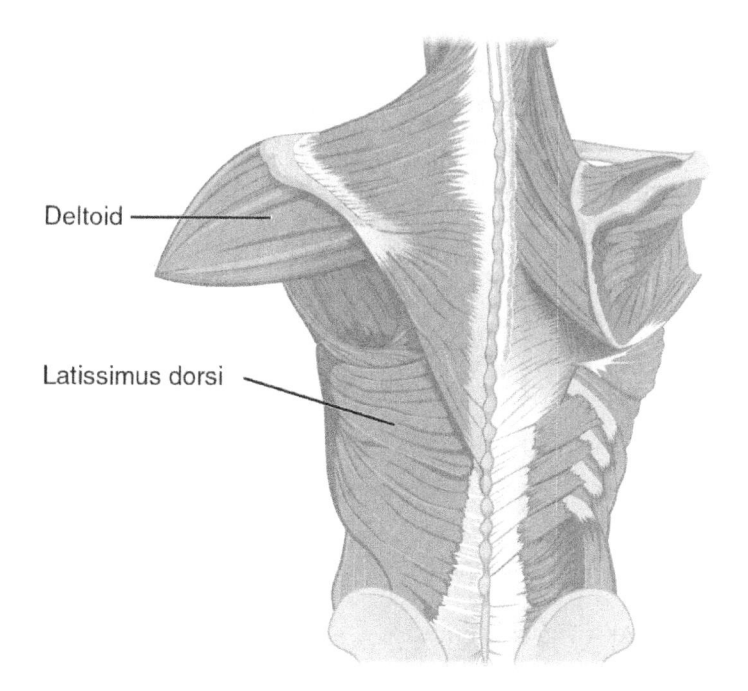

The latissimus dorsi muscles work with the chest muscles or the pectoralis major to help the body rotate and, therefore, the golf swing.

The pectoralis major extends from the sternum at the mid-point of the chest up to the shoulder on each side of the body.

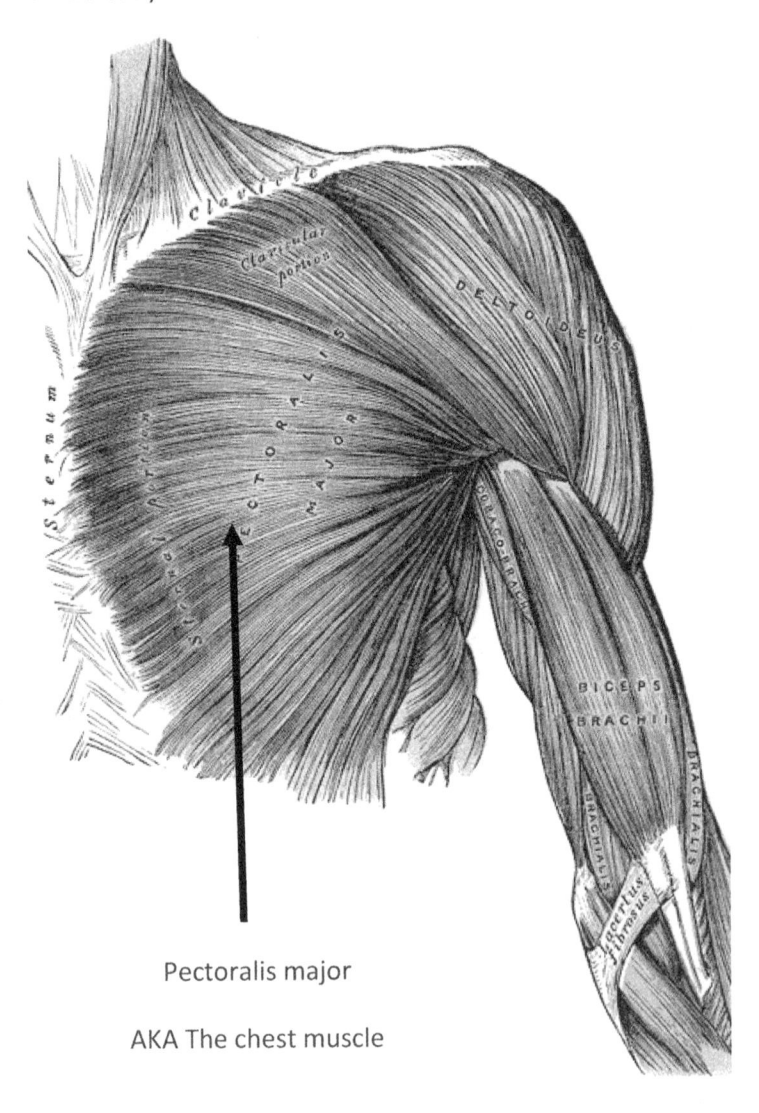

Pectoralis major

AKA The chest muscle

The shoulder muscles are extremely important to the golf swing and help to generate speed and maintain control. The ball and socket shoulder joint are extraordinarily complex, as are the myriad of muscles surrounding it. However, the primary deltoid or shoulder muscles involved are the anterior (front) deltoid, the lateral (side) deltoid, and the posterior (rear) deltoid.

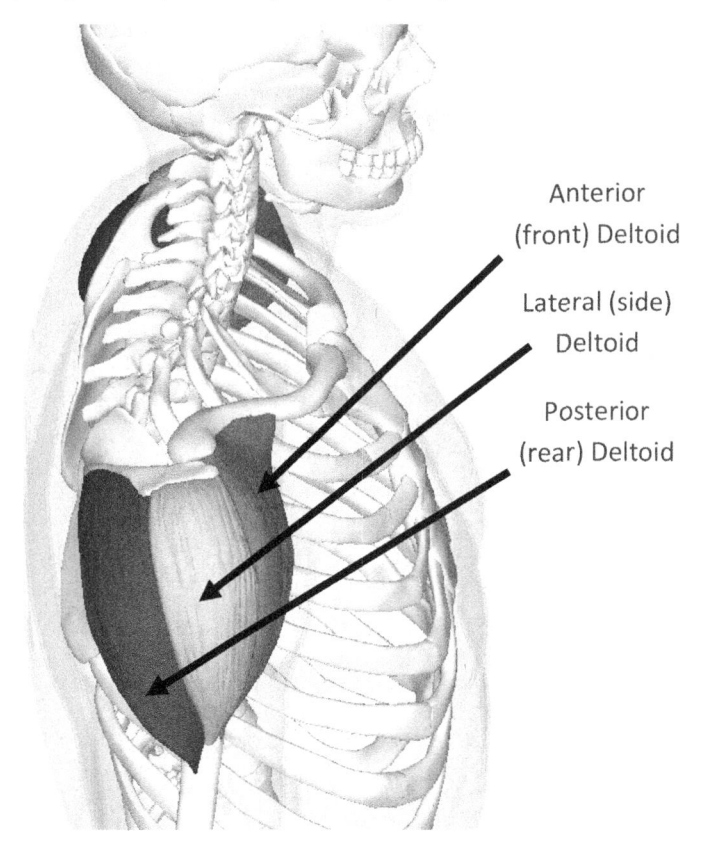

Anterior (front) Deltoid

Lateral (side) Deltoid

Posterior (rear) Deltoid

Last but certainly not least, the legs and buttocks are another vital anatomical component of a good golf swing. The legs provide a solid base posture for everything else to function. The gluteus maximus, AKA the buttocks, helps in the ability to rotate and work with the thighs to provide solid lower body support. The slightly bent knee stance during a golf swing engages the quadriceps, AKA the front thigh muscles, and in turn, works in conjunction with the calf muscles and buttocks. Keeping the buttocks tight before and during a swing will help keep the lower body still and provide the solid foundation needed for the entire swing duration.

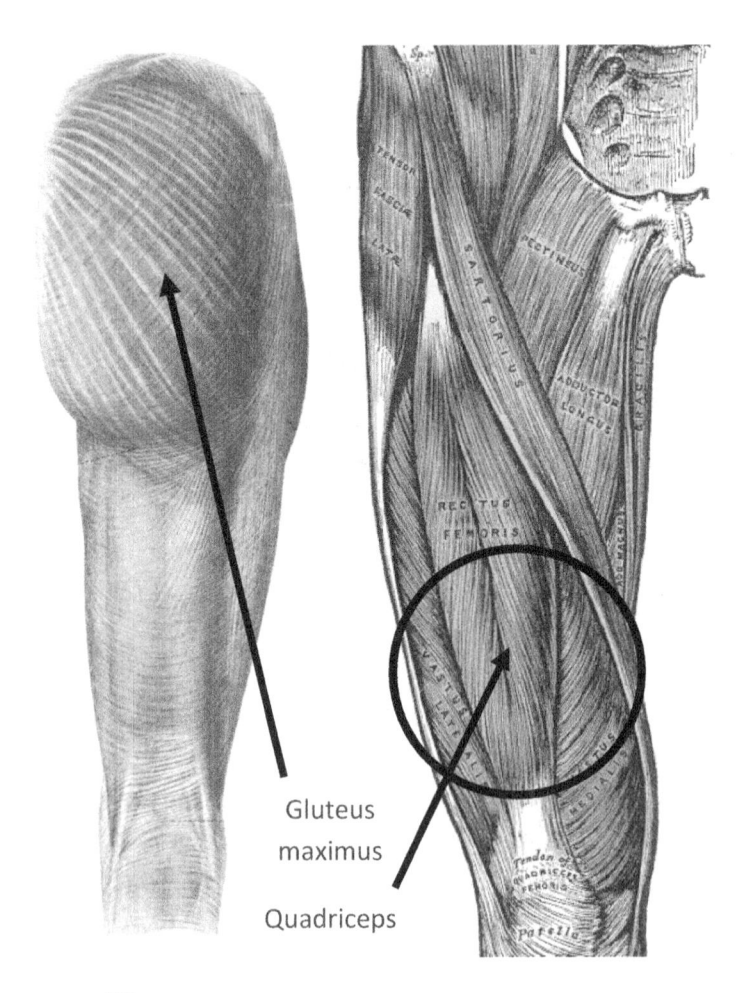

Gluteus maximus

Quadriceps

A Golfer's Walk is a Healthy Walk

It is just a fact that a lot of walking is involved during a golf practice session or when playing a game of golf. Leaving aside any other physical aspect of the game, just the walking aspect can have enormous health benefits.

In the journal Healthy Heart for Life!, Dr Martha Grogan of Mayo Clinic in Rochester, Minnesota, said that research indicates that walking for just 10 minutes daily can halve one's risk of a heart attack. She also said that a sedentary lifestyle increases the risk of a heart attack almost as much as smoking does.

Therefore, given that golf typically involves walking for far longer than just 10 minutes a day, golfers are dramatically reducing their risk of a heart attack while simultaneously having fun.

In Great Britain, the NHS research indicates the same as the Mayo Clinic research. After the results of an extensive international study were published, the NHS highly recommends walking as an excellent exercise that helps prevent several serious illnesses and diseases.

Other studies focussed on adults at high risk of type 2 diabetes and heart disease. Research has found that an additional 2,000 steps per day lowered the risk of experiencing a cardiac issue by up to 10% for this group of people. Furthermore, continuing research indicated that for every additional 2,000 steps per day taken, the risk is further reduced by 8%.

The research was carried out by teams from the NIHR Leicester-Loughborough Diet, Lifestyle, and Physical

Activity Biomedical Research Unit, the University of Leicester, and Duke University School of Medicine in the USA. They also collaborated with other researchers from universities and institutes around the world. The results were published in the medical journal The Lancet.

Research also indicates that two and a half hours of walking each week can help to reduce the risk of contracting seven types of cancer. The research suggested that increasing the length of time spent walking/taking moderate exercise to five hours per week reduced the risk of kidney cancer in both sexes by 11 per cent and 17 per cent, respectively.

The research also suggested that two and a half hours of walking each week could reduce the risk of contracting breast cancer by 5% and by 10% for five hours of walking per week. Women were up to 18% less likely to get cancer of the womb, both sexes were less likely to get non-Hodgkin's lymphoma, up to 19 per cent less likely to contract myeloma, and men were up to 14% less likely to get colon cancer. The details of the study were published in the Journal of Clinical Oncology.

Golf Clubs - Overview

Since even those who are new to golf will know the typical technical construction overview of the average set of golf clubs, what is the ideal type of club to use as an IIED or Improvised Isometric Exercise Device?

The best type is always going to be the strongest one. It affords the user the best overall grip when both ends of the shaft are held and is the best balanced with the lightest head. A lighter head is always going to work best as an IIED or Improvised Isometric Exercise Device because it will be the easiest to use and remain in a balanced position during the majority of isometric exercises.

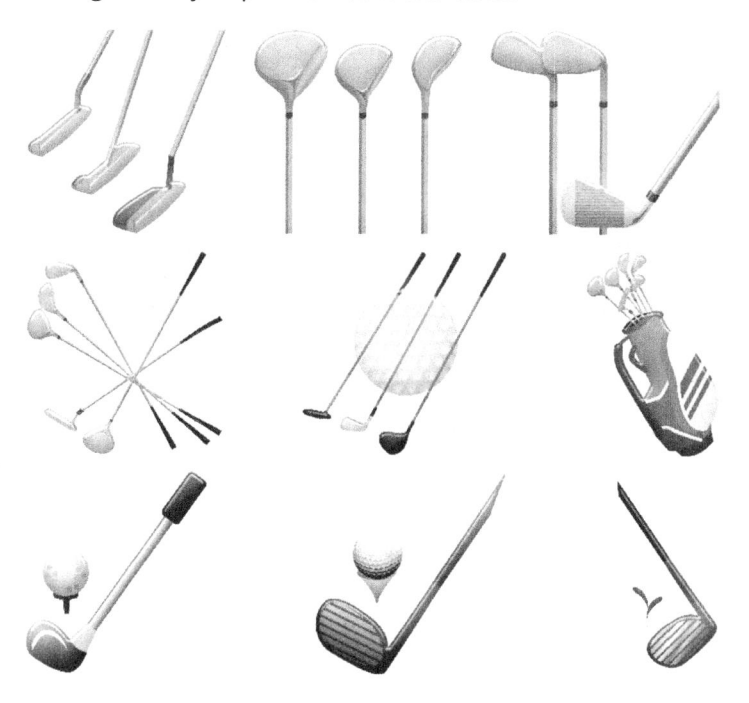

Therefore, the best type of club to use is probably a simple putter. As a note of caution, the shaft may always become permanently very slightly distorted during an isometric exercise.

This is never usually a problem with higher-quality golf clubs. However, if you are a strong person who is going to exercise regularly, as suggested, then you may wish to dedicate an old golf club specifically for the heavier type of exercise. For the rest of us who are not able to bend metal bars, this should never be an issue.

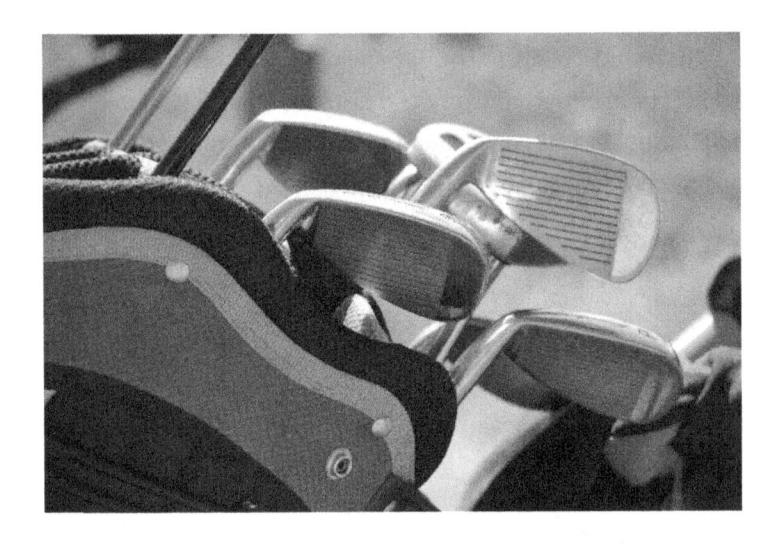

Golfer's Elbow

Medial epicondylitis is the technical medical term for what is better known as golfer's elbow. This injury causes pain and inflammation primarily through overusing the muscles and tendons that connect the forearm to the elbow.

This is because any action that enables one to grip, flex the wrist, and rotate the arm can, through repeated action, cause microtrauma/tiny tears in the tendons. The pain is typically centred on and around the inside of the elbow, where the protruding lump of bone is. However, it may also radiate into the forearm.

Golfer's elbow is technically the less well-known relative of tennis elbow, and they are both forms of tendonitis. The difference between the two is that golfer's elbow tends to be caused by microtrauma to the tendons on the inside of the elbow, whereas tennis elbow stems from damage to tendons on the outside.

Typically, golfer's elbow is related to the flexor muscles in the forearm. These muscles enable one to close the fingers into a curved gripping position and also help bend the palm/fist/wrist inward.

The muscles and tendons are designed to perform these actions, so they are no problem under normal circumstances. However, microtrauma becomes an issue when the normal action of the flexor muscles is interfered with in some way.

Surprisingly to many, golfer's elbow is a problem that does not only affect golfers. This is because any kind of repetitive hand/wrist/forearm motion/use can lead to developing similar problems.

Similar issues can be caused by microtrauma from repetitive strain when using tools such as a screwdriver, a hammer, or even a paintbrush. Many sports, particularly ball-throwing games such as cricket and baseball, can also cause similar issues.

Interestingly, golfers' and tennis elbows are part of what is commonly known as Bullworker® elbow. The Bullworker® is the classic isotonic/isometric exercise device that was first launched in the 1960s. It is still a best-seller even today for a simple reason: It works.

However, some people occasionally develop what has become known as *Bullworker® elbow* due to incorrect use of the device in certain exercises, primarily chest compression. It has nothing to do with the device itself; it is all about the user's lack of attention to detail when following the instructions.

How does one prevent golfer's elbow? There are several ways to do this, and they primarily include identifying and eliminating all obvious sources of strain, which will dramatically decrease the risk of creating microtrauma damage. Also, it is important to always follow the correct biomechanical action/form when playing golf or any other sport or physical activity.

This is an excellent reason why people first learning how to play golf should get expert coaching from a professional coach so that bad techniques and habits can be eliminated from the start. Also, when gripping objects, ensure that you do so in a biomechanically efficient way with the wrist level, and aligned with the forearm.

Stretching can help, too. All stretching should be performed slowly because aggressive stretching will only aggravate any problems you have. The best stretches to perform are ones that lengthen the flexor muscles of the forearm by bending your wrist or fingers toward the back of your hand; you can also reverse the action.

If you are unlucky enough to contract golfer's elbow, then it is always best to seek professional medical treatment from your doctor. However, you can always help the treatment/rehabilitation process by resting the affected area and by applying regular ice packs to reduce inflammation.

Most sports professionals will immediately apply an icepack if they are unlucky enough to sustain an injury of some kind. Research indicates that the sooner an icepack can be applied to the injured area, the better. Early application and then regular re-application of icepacks to a strain/injury have been shown to reduce the recovery time needed dramatically.

When it comes to treating injuries, sports professionals use the acronym R.I.C.E., which stands for Rest, Ice, Compression, and Elevation. This process reduces inflammation/swelling, provides certain pain relief, and reduces the recovery time needed to typically only a few days or weeks.

When it comes to preventing golfer's elbow, the stronger the muscles and tendons, the less likely they are to become injured in the first place.

A strain injury occurs because the action being performed has found a weakness, and if the muscles and tendons were stronger, then a strain would be much less likely to occur.

Therefore, a regular strength training programme such as the one outlined in this book will help you develop much stronger muscles and tendons, which will directly reduce your risk of developing golfer's elbow.

Chapter 2:
Exercise Science Overview

In this chapter, we will give a user-friendly overview of exercise science together with the features and benefits of various exercise techniques and concepts. For those who want more in-depth information about the science of isometric exercise and health and fitness in general, then we suggest that you also read our books The ISOmetric Bible™ and The 70 Second Difference™ books. Both are available on Amazon.

Walking as Exercise

Walking is a vastly underrated form of exercise; even a short, regular daily walk can yield tremendous health benefits. In recent years, several notable studies have been performed on the health-related benefits of walking and how walking can even help prevent many serious diseases and illnesses.

In the journal Healthy Heart for Life!, Dr Martha Grogan of the Mayo Clinic in Rochester, Minnesota, said that research indicates that walking for just 10 minutes a day can halve one's risk of having a heart attack. She also said that a sedentary lifestyle increases the risk of a heart attack almost as much as smoking does.

Therefore, given that golf typically involves walking far longer than just 10 minutes a day, even golfers are dramatically cutting their risk of a heart attack while simultaneously having fun. Whereas Nordic Walkers and Trekkers naturally gain even greater health-related benefits due to the greater distances they walk.

In Great Britain, the NHS research indicates the same as the Mayo Clinic research. After the results of an extensive international study were published, the National Health Service highly recommends walking as an excellent form of exercise that helps to prevent several serious illnesses and diseases.

Other studies focussed on adults with a high risk of type 2 diabetes and heart disease. Research has found that an additional 2,000 steps per day lowered the risk of experiencing a cardiac issue by up to 10% for this group of people. Furthermore, continuing research indicated that for every additional 2,000 steps per day that were taken, it further reduced the risk by 8%. The research was carried out by teams from the NIHR Leicester-Loughborough Diet, Lifestyle, and Physical Activity Biomedical Research Unit, the University of Leicester, and Duke University School of Medicine in the USA. They also collaborated with other researchers from universities and institutes around the world. The results were published in the medical journal The Lancet.

Research indicates that two and a half hours of walking each week can also help to reduce the risk of contracting seven types of cancer. The research suggested that it reduced the risk of kidney cancer in both sexes by 11 per cent and by 17 per cent if the length of time spent walking/taking moderate exercise was increased to five hours per week. The research also suggested that two and a half hours of walking each week could reduce the risk of contracting breast cancer by 5% and by 10% for five hours of walking per week. Women were up to 18% less likely to get cancer of the womb, both sexes were less likely to get non-Hodgkin's lymphoma, up to 19 per cent less likely to contract myeloma, and men were up to 14% less likely to get colon cancer. The details of the study were published in the Journal of Clinical Oncology.

Walking Vs Running as a Fat Burner

Walking and running are both excellent ways to get fitter, burn calories, tone up, and promote weight loss. There are different and distinct benefits to each, which we will briefly touch on. Running burns more calories than walking does. However, walking burns more fat than running does. So, it is a trade-off, especially since walking more will increase your N.E.A.T. factor. We will explain more about N.E.A.T. in the next section.

When exercising at a lower intensity, fat is used as the body's primary fuel. When you shift gears and increase the pace from walking to running, your body burns more carbohydrates as fuel.

However, it does not matter too much whether you are burning body fat or carbohydrates as the primary fuel. What is important is that you burn the most calories possible during your exercise session and stimulate a long-term increase in your Base Metabolic Rate. Therefore, even though walking may burn more stored fat as fuel, running will still burn more overall calories.

Another important factor to consider when looking at the differences between walking and running is the risk of injury from each. Running carries more risk of injury than walking, so the choice is yours.

Walking, General Activity and N.E.A.T. - Non-Exercise Activity Thermogenesis

The acronym N.E.A.T. is becoming increasingly discussed in relation to weight control, body fat, and exercise. The N.E.A.T. acronym stands for Non-Exercise Activity Thermogenesis, and it comes from Dr James Levine's research into how we expend calories. In simple terms, it means: "burning calories through daily life, and not through exercise," and in the simplest terms, it means that people who are active and move around a lot burn more calories and tend to be slimmer than people who do not.

There are two basic ways in which we burn calories. One is while we exercise, and the other is through the general activities of daily living. The key question is: "Which, if any, is more important to weight loss, and the levels of body fat that we carry?" According to Dr Levine, it is the N.E.A.T. that appears to be far more important for calorie burning than dedicated exercise time. Dr Levine's research also led to the phrase: "Being Active Naturally" becoming more commonly used.

Providing that you exercise good judgement in your food choices and the macros around proper portion control, in addition to your regular exercise routine, just being a little more active in everyday life will make a huge difference in terms of weight control and overall body fat levels.

In our opinion, N.E.A.T. alone is not a great panacea when it comes to losing weight and staying slim. After all, when people are stressed and mentally fatigued because of a tough workday, it is not always easy to opt for the most sensible food choices, nor is it likely that you will want to go out and do something active to increase your daily movement factor. However, N.E.A.T. is certainly something to be factored into your overall lifestyle because it makes a significant difference to your overall appearance and fitness levels.

The Basic Types of Resistance Exercise

All muscle training falls into two or three specific categories, depending on how you break them down. In the most basic form, there are two types: contraction with or without movement. Breaking them down a step further, there become three categories, with one being isotonic, another isokinetic, and last but certainly not least, isometric.

Isotonic training is all about movement, with muscle shortening and lengthening during the lifting and lowering phases of the exercise. We know that the isotonic category can be broken down further into three parts. One part is the concentric contraction, which is the lifting phase of an exercise when the muscles shorten. Another is the eccentric phase, the lowering part of an exercise when the muscles lengthen.

Lastly, the isotonic category includes the isokinetic contraction. In this contraction, the muscle changes in length during both the concentric and eccentric phases; however, the velocity remains constant no matter how much force is applied during the exercises.

Then comes the isometric category. With an isometric exercise, there is no movement whatsoever. To help you envision this, I will take a random weight training or freehand callisthenic exercise, such as a chest press because it can be performed either with movement OR without movement as an isometric exercise.

For example, a barbell, a machine, or your bodyweight can be lifted and lowered to perform an exercise such as a barbell curl. This is called isotonic exercise, callisthenics, or simply exercise with movement.

To perform the same or similar exercise isometrically, you would attempt to perform the same or similar biomechanically correct actions of a barbell curl. However, at a certain point, or points if multiple exercise points were being used, the curling movement would stop because an immovable object point had been reached.

At that point or points, you would apply an increasing level of force until you reach the desired target level as you attempt to perform the curling exercise against the immovable object.

At the desired isometric exercise point, a constant force is applied against the immovable object for 7 seconds, which is the optimum isometric exercise time. The ideal basic isometric exercise point for general exercise is roughly at the mid-point when your muscles reach a stalemate working against each other or an immovable object. This is called a Standard isometric Contraction.

The harder you engage your muscles as you try to break the stalemate by lifting, pushing, or pulling, the stronger your muscles become. In doing so, you engage many more muscle fibres than normal as you attempt to move the immovable object and perform the curling exercise action.

Doors, desks, chairs, walls, and many other everyday items can serve as immovable objects. However, the simplest and most accessible immovable object is often yourself, making isometric exercise a convenient and empowering choice.

Isometric Overview

As you now know, isometric exercise does not involve any movement. Instead, the joint angle and the muscle length do not change during contraction. You also now know that 7 seconds is regarded as the optimum time to perform an isometric exercise.

However, almost everyone tends to count the exercise elapsed time much faster than the real elapsed time when exercising. This means that it is easy not to reach the magic 7 seconds of the optimum isometric exercise time. Therefore, we always suggest aiming to perform the exercise for 10 seconds to ensure that the 7-second target is always reached, even when under the stress of intense exercise.

Isometric exercise has been extensively scientifically researched and repeatedly proven to be a highly effective method for building strength and muscle. It is one of the most thoroughly researched exercise systems despite being one of the most misunderstood. This is likely due to fear, professional ignorance, and financial reasons, but the evidence of its effectiveness is undeniable.

The isometric exercise system can use several different techniques. Most of these techniques are highly advanced and intended for competitive athletes, martial arts practitioners, strength athletes, and bodybuilders. Therefore, they are not appropriate for a general isometric exercise session for the average person who simply wants to get stronger and fitter.

However, purely out of interest, I will list them here in case any fitness enthusiasts, athletes, or bodybuilders read this book and wish to try them. They are described in greater detail in our book called The Isometric Bible which is available on Amazon and in good bookstores. The most common and advanced isometric exercise techniques include the following:

- Standard Isometric Contraction
- Yielding Isometric Contraction
- Maximum Duration Isometrics
- Oscillatory Isometrics
- Impact Absorption Isometrics
- Explosive Isometrics, AKA: Ballistic Isometrics
- Static-Dynamic Isometric
- Contrast Isometric
- Functional Isometrics
- TRISOmetrics™

More than enough isometric exercises can be performed without any equipment to allow a total body workout routine to be completed relatively easily. These will typically be self-resisted isometric exercises, which are excellent. However, by using only minimal readily available equipment such as walking poles, golf clubs, martial arts belts, climbing ropes, scuba diving webbing weight belts, and broom handles, etc., it is possible to greatly expand the number of exercises that can be performed.

It is also perfectly possible to adapt and use other readily available items such as tow ropes, steel chains, towels, and commonly found immobile objects such as sturdy fixed barrier railings, solid walls, solid doors, door frames, or parked vehicles to perform a complete isometric exercise routine. Again, these are all excellent improvised exercise tools that allow an expanded range of highly effective isometric exercises to be performed.

Using improvised exercise tools can yield an unexpected additional benefit. This is because it allows one to focus more and apply greater concentration to each exercise. This is particularly useful for those who are either completely new to or are relatively new to the isometric exercise system. We will explain more about what these can be later in the book.

One of the things we love about both the isometric and self-resisted systems of exercise is that as you get stronger through exercise, you can apply more force and intensity to your isometric or self-resisted exercises.

This, in turn, means that you can gradually increase the level of force and intensity you can safely apply to each exercise which will mean that the results and benefits you receive will grow in a compound way through regular daily use. This is what we call a natural Adaptive Response™ mechanism, which is a useful aspect of our biology.

Isometric Exercise Science

Even until the mid-20th century, almost no scientific research had been performed into the benefits of isometric exercise. We also know that before the first serious scientific research study, people trained isometrically by performing what we now call endurance isometrics.

Thankfully, isometric exercise has been thoroughly scientifically researched and proven for several decades. I would estimate that at least as much scientific research has been performed on it as on traditional resistance training.

The first major in-depth study into isometric exercise was performed at the world-famous Max Plank Institute in Dortmund, Germany. If you already have a reasonable knowledge of science, you will also know that the Max Plank Institute is a world-renowned centre of scientific excellence in many disciplines.

Between 1953 and 1958, one of the most extensive research studies was commissioned into isometric exercise science. These experiments are now considered by many to be the original gold standard of isometric exercise studies. The results were made widespread public knowledge in the resultant ground-breaking book, The Physiology of Strength, by Dr Theodor Hettinger - Research Fellow at the Max Plank Institute. During that 5-year research period, Dr Hettinger and Dr Muller performed a widely reported, reputed 5,500 experiments, although this figure is almost certainly apocryphal because they would have had to perform a minimum of three experiments a day, every day for five years. Research suggests that the number of experiments Hettinger and Muller performed was probably closer to 200.

However, in wider studies at other institutions since that time, over 5,500 studies have almost certainly been completed. These were conducted on male and female volunteers from all walks of life and at every level of strength, fitness, and athletic ability. Perhaps what surprised people the most was how dramatic and impressive the results were gained from performing isometric exercises. Also, because the same or similar results were easily repeatable, the data gained from the experiments was exceptionally reliable. The conclusion of the extensive studies proved beyond doubt the overall superiority of isometric exercise in building strength and muscle compared to traditional isotonic exercise methods. It also proved that the isometric system delivered these results much faster and with far less exercise than traditional resistance training.

Another extremely interesting result emerged from the experiments. This was because the optimum results were not produced by the length of time an isometric exercise was held but by the correct level of force applied for a specific optimum time.

They found that performing only one daily isometric exercise for between just 6 and 7 seconds, and at only two-thirds of an individual's maximum effort, could increase strength by an average of up to 5% per week. By any standards, strength gains of 5% in exchange for the expenditure of only 66%, or around two-thirds of an individual's maximum capacity, is an excellent result.

Perhaps even more amazingly, they discovered that after someone has performed a single 7-second training stimulus (exercise) per day, the muscle being exercised in that same position was no longer responsive to further gains. In other words, it did not matter how many more times you exercised the same muscle in the same position; there would be no further increase in muscle growth or strength. The only way to do this was to perform another isometric exercise at a different position, only the limb's ROM (Range Of Motion). The scientific data about this can be referenced on pages 28 to 31 of Dr Theodor Hettinger's book, "The Physiology of Strength."

In 2001, Nicolas Babault, PhD of the University of Burgundy, Dijon, France, led a team of scientists to research and examine how many muscle fibres were activated and how long they remained active during both traditional weight training and isometric training.

(*The scientific research paper is published: Nicolas Babault, Michel Pousson, Yves Ballay, and Jacques Van Hoecke - Groupe Analyse du Mouvement, Unité de Formation et de Recherche Sciences et Techniques des Activités Physiques et Sportives, Université de Bourgogne, BP 27877, 21078 Dijon Cedex, France.*)

They discovered that when training intensely and in near-perfect style, the levels of muscle activation during repetitions of optimum maximal weight training were between 89.7% during the concentric contraction, or when lifting a weight, and 88.3% during the eccentric contraction, or when lowering a weight. For practical purposes, an average of about 89% overall.

The study also revealed that during the lifting, or concentric part of the exercise, the maximum intramuscular tension only lasted for between 0.25 and 0.5 seconds. Which, for practical purposes is an average of about 1/3rd of a second during each isotonic repetition. This is because traditional isotonic resistance exercises naturally involve movement. They also have aspects of velocity and acceleration to consider in the overall equation. "Force" is only produced for a split second to produce a maximal contraction of the muscle fibres. The same research also showed that the level of muscle activation during isometric exercise was as high as 95.2% and that it lasted for the entire 7 to 10 seconds of each exercise. This is a huge increase over the 1/3rd of a second muscular activation achieved during a single repetition of weight training.

Therefore, based on these discoveries, technically, a single isometric exercise performed at only two-thirds of an individual's maximum can deliver similar or often even better results than the equivalent of up to 3 sets of 10 weight training repetitions in the lifting phase of the exercise.

To explain this further, I will use a typical barbell curl exercise in the lifting phase as my example, where the object of the exercise is to engage as many muscle fibres as possible in a maximum muscular contraction. Naturally, 3 sets of 10 repetitions give us an overall total of 30 repetitions. One set of 10 repetitions of the barbell curl in perfect high-intensity style produces a maximum muscular engagement for approximately 3.3 seconds. Three sets of 10 repetitions of the same exercise, a total of 30 repetitions, will give a total of approximately 9.9 seconds of maximum muscular engagement and an average of 89% muscle activation overall.

In comparison, one high-intensity isometric contraction exercise produces a maximum muscular engagement that lasts for the entire duration of the exercise. Even though the optimum time over which an isometric exercise is performed was found to be 7 seconds, this is almost always rounded up to the 10-second target number. The maximum muscular engagement will last for the entire 10 seconds of a high-intensity isometric exercise with 95.2% muscle activation overall.

This is proof that is based entirely on scientific research that 3 sets of 10 near-perfect high-intensity curls when weight training, which takes several minutes to perform, still was not quite equal to the results achieved by a single 10-second high-intensity isometric curl exercise.

The Standard Isometric Contraction

The standard isometric contraction is a simple and highly effective technique. Therefore, this is the technique we will focus on for practical isometric training.

The standard isometric contraction, AKA: overcoming isometric contraction, AKA: maximum-effort isometrics, or whatever else you wish to call it, is when a muscle is applying force to push or pull against an immovable resistance. This is the most basic of all kinds of isometric exercise, and it is highly effective. This type of isometric contraction exercise was performed during the experiments by Dr T. Hettinger and Dr E. Muller at the Max Plank Institute. It is also the technique referred to in their book The Physiology of Strength.

In a standard isometric contraction, it is theoretically possible to exert up to 100% of one's maximum capacity effort against an immovable object and then continue to hold that level of force throughout the exercise. This means that standard isometric contraction can be a very high-intensity exercise system.

Performing an isometric exercise against an immovable object at a certain level of force for a given duration of time will teach your body to recruit more muscle fibres to try to move the object. As you perform the exercise and generate as much force as possible, your CNS, or Central Nervous System, learns that it needs to activate and recruit more muscle fibres to reach the goal of moving the object.

Since this will naturally be impossible to move, the process will continue each time you exercise to make you stronger and grow more muscle. Your body mechanisms become trained to readily activate and recruit additional muscle fibres when facing similar challenges, which, in turn, repeats the cycle more readily every time.

As we mentioned earlier, the immovable/solid object can be anything completely solid and safe to use. This can be a wall, a door, a door jamb, a parked motor vehicle or anything similar. Perhaps the most common objects used to enhance everyday isometric exercise training are sturdy towels, climbing ropes, martial arts belts, scuba diving weight belts, webbing straps, golf clubs, and broom handles etc. All the aforementioned items are excellent when used properly and will deliver some excellent results. More importantly, they are typically readily available for most people, which makes exercising with them so much easier.

Another common way to perform isometric exercise is to do it in a self-resisted way. Self-resisting means pushing or pulling against your limbs/hands/feet, etc. For example, you might place the palms of your hands together at chest level with your hands roughly at the midpoint of your body. In that position, you would then press your hands together using your chest muscles to provide the primary driving force, then you are performing a highly effective self-resisted isometric chest press!

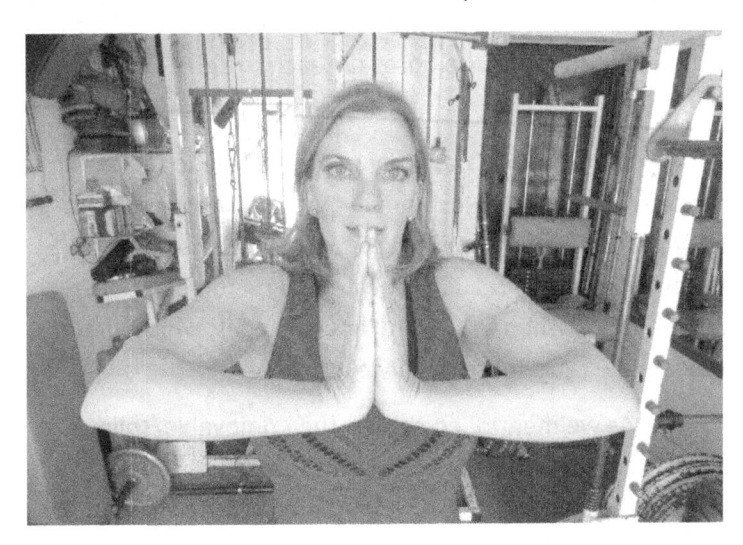

It is possible to perform a well-balanced and highly effective self-resisted isometric workout to exercise virtually every section of the body. So, never underestimate self-resisted exercise because it can be immensely powerful indeed. Also, self-resistance exercises are an excellent way to ensure that a personal maximum resistance is used safely and with minimum risk of injury caused by applying too much force.

The fact is that it does not matter which method is chosen. It can be isometrics performed against an immovable object, self-resisted isometrics, or a combination of the two. The most important thing is that either the object must be completely immovable through human muscle power alone, or the force of one body part must be able to completely counterbalance the force of another body part to produce a muscular stalemate.

Intensity, Force, Strength, and Power

Intensity will always be a relative term, and it is often completely misunderstood when used regarding exercise. When it comes to exercising your muscles, intensity is the percentage of your ability to move a resistance. Technically, an individual's highest possible level of intensity is when they reach a point of momentary failure after exerting themselves completely.

However, the important questions we need to try to answer are: "How hard is hard?" and "How intense is intense?" To some degree, both are very subjective. Taking two people of roughly equal fitness, something that is intense to one person might be considered comparatively easy to the other.

Hard is a relative term, and handling 50 lbs of resistance is impossibly hard if your strength is only at the level required to lift 49 lbs. However, if you can lift 100 lbs as a maximum, then lifting 50 lbs is going to be comparatively easy.

Often, the only factors differentiating between people and the intensity level exerted are mental toughness, determination, and perception.

Therefore, to gain the greatest benefits from isometric exercise, the first thing that must be learned is how to determine, with a reasonable degree of accuracy, what level of intensity is being applied to an exercise.

It is just a fact that what one person deems to be 100% of their capacity will always be quite different from another person's estimate. The accurate estimation of what one person deems to be 2/3rds of their overall maximum intensity will also vary from person to person. The accuracy of estimation will also vary greatly between an experienced professional athlete and an absolute beginner to exercise.

Experience has taught us that most people who are new to exercise will always fall well short of accurately estimating any given percentage. A beginner will find it more challenging to accurately estimate what 2/3rds of their 100% maximum is compared to a more experienced athlete. Many people might believe they are performing at 100% capacity when they are only performing at around 2/3rds, or perhaps at only 50% or less of their 100% maximum.

This is because exercise is new to them, and therefore, the experiences and feelings in their bodies associated with it are also new. They simply have no common frame of reference when it comes to calculating/estimating their level of physical exertion.

The human brain has a built-in mechanism that helps to protect the body and prevent it from performing a physical activity to such a level that it could cause serious damage or even death. This is the mechanism that makes your brain tell you to stop exercising when it begins to get tough, and the feeling of wanting to stop exercising only increases as you continue to push yourself harder to do more. This is all despite the biological fact that you are physically capable of doing much more than is being suggested by the messages you are receiving from yourself.

Over time, the brains of people who exercise regularly, especially to high intensity, will naturally adjust and reposition this built-in safety margin. This means that the brain of an experienced high-level athlete does not "tell" them to stop an exercise until the level of intensity is much higher than it would be for a beginner.

Therefore, how is it possible to subjectively quantify and then impart appropriate levels of recommended intensity when it comes to exercise? This problem is even more challenging when one considers that accurately translating and subjectively assessing various intensity levels will always be subjective to every individual.

If you were to train as hard as humanly possible, with near 100% maximum intensity, which involves super-strict form and training to complete failure and beyond, then you simply could not train for a long time. It is just physiologically impossible. Physics and biology are quite simple in this respect.

The intensity of your workout is directly proportional to the length of time you can physically perform it. The harder and more intensely you exercise, the shorter the time you can physically perform it.

Make no mistake, performing a 7-second isometric exercise while exerting close to your personal 100% maximum physical capacity is completely and utterly exhausting, even for a professional athlete.

What does all this mean when it comes to accurately communicating various levels of exercise intensity, especially when there is no professional coach or elaborate and expensive measuring equipment at hand?

Research clearly shows that almost everyone will stop exercising long before they are in any danger of becoming seriously fatigued. Most people will *think* they are exercising at a much higher intensity than they would if they were only a little more mentally resilient.

This does not mean that people should suddenly begin pushing themselves beyond their physical limits, which would be stupid. However, it does mean that most people who enjoy a higher-than-average level of mental resilience, determination, and being in physically good condition can push themselves much harder than they might think. If anyone ever feels "genuine" strain or fatigue to the point of becoming injured, then they should stop exercising immediately.

Even without the aid of a professional coach to monitor, encourage you, and measure your intensity and progress with specialist equipment, the tips we have outlined in this section will help you get the most out of every workout. It is also worth remembering that if you cheat, then the only person who loses is you.

As a footnote, for the sake of clarification, exercise intensity refers to how much energy is expended when exercising, including the amount of weight used per repetition. Perceived intensity varies with each person. Intensity and force are technically different but are frequently accepted as interchangeable terms in the common vernacular.

Muscular strength is different from muscular endurance, which is the ability to produce and sustain muscle force over a certain period of time. While strength is the maximum force you can apply against a load, power is proportional to the speed at which you can explosively apply it. In other words, it is the ability to quickly produce a given amount of force.

Muscular force, often referred to as muscular strength, is the physical power exerted by muscles to perform various actions, such as lifting, pushing, or pulling objects. It results from the contraction of muscles and is vital for human mobility and functionality.

Technically, How Does a Muscle Grow?

How does a muscle grow? This is one of the most common questions concerning fitness and exercise. However, it is also one of the most misunderstood concepts, even amongst fitness professionals and personal trainers. To see for yourself just how uninformed or badly informed some people are, simply join one or two of the social media groups online so you can read some of the absolute drivel posted by 'keyboard warriors' who purport to be 'experts' on the subject. Alarmingly, many of these people seem to have developed a hardcore following, which to the science-based professional is like watching 'fools leading other fools' on a wild goose chase.

So, back to the key question which is, how does a muscle grow? To explain this, we must examine three concepts: 1) muscle growth through increases in the volume/size of myofibrils inside the muscles, commonly called myofibrillar hypertrophy. 2) hyperplasia, which is when there is an increase in the number of muscle cells/fibres. 3) sarcoplasmic growth, which is all about increasing the fluid content.

When it comes to exercise, the muscles you wish to grow must be challenged with a workload greater than they can currently accommodate. In other words, an exercise that is intense enough to stimulate growth. This stimulus can come from any source such as lifting a heavy object, weight training, isometrics, compressing a spring in a device such as a Bullworker™, or through self-resistance either hand to hand or limb to limb or using an Iso-Bow™ etc.

This process creates trauma to the muscle fibres, disrupting the muscle cell organelles. This then triggers other cells outside the muscle fibres to greatly increase in numbers at and around the point of the trauma to repair the damage. The process of repair involves a fusion of cells. This, in turn, causes the cross-sectional area of the muscle fibre to increase because the muscle cell myofibrils increase in both size and quantity. This process is more commonly known as hypertrophy. Since this process increases the number of cellular nuclei, the muscle fibres generate more myosin and actin. These are contractile protein myofilaments, which help make the muscle stronger.

This is the basis of what is more commonly known as myofibril muscle growth. In addition to this, there is also probably a process called hyperplasia which takes place. I use the term 'probably' because this concept is extremely controversial for many reasons. One of the key problems is that evidence of this in human beings is lacking, whereas there is a mass of evidence supporting hyperplasia in mice and other animals.

Hypertrophy is the increase in the size of the existing muscle fibres to accommodate the increased demands placed upon them through intense exercise. Hyperplasia, concerning skeletal muscle growth, is the increase in the number of muscle fibres, which in turn will also increase the cross-sectional area of a muscle.

Despite a lack of evidence supporting hyperplasia in human beings, logic supports the process. This is because of a theory known as Nuclear Domain Theory. This states that the nucleus of a cell (a muscle cell in this instance) is only able to control a finite area of cellular space. It is thought that satellite cells donate their nuclei to the muscle cell until a certain point is reached when this can no longer take place.

Beyond a certain limit, and through continued intense training, the cell must eventually divide to create two cells instead of the former single cell. When this happens, the entire hypertrophy process starts over once again. This probably means that most of the muscle growth is almost certainly caused by hypertrophy, and a much smaller percentage can be attributed to hyperplasia at any given point in the muscle stimulus/growth process.

Finally, there is the subject of sarcoplasmic muscle growth to address. Sarcoplasmic muscle growth is the increase in the volume of sarcoplasmic fluid in the muscle cell. These fluids and energy resources surround the myofibrils in your muscles, containing mostly glycogen together with other elements, including creatine, ATP, and water.

To clarify, glycogen is simply a type of sugar that serves as a form of energy. It is deposited in bodily tissues as a store of carbohydrates, and it is the body's main form of storage for the sugar glucose. Glycogen is stored in two main places in the body, one being the liver and the other being the muscles.

More importantly, glycogen is the body's secondary source of long-term energy storage, with fat being the primary energy storage source. When glycogen is in the muscles, it is converted into glucose for use as energy when performing sports, etc., and glycogen stored in the liver is converted into glucose for use as energy throughout the body and in the central nervous system.

Therefore, sarcoplasmic growth increases muscle volume, but this increase is not in functional strength mass since it does not increase the number of muscle fibres. It is like 'the pump' in that it increases the size and shape of the muscle through the muscle holding an increased amount of fluid.

Rest Time Between Exercises

Naturally, the rest time between exercises during a workout is quite different from the rest and recovery needed to allow your body to respond positively to the stimulus generated by exercise.

If you keep the rest time between exercises brief enough, the workout routine itself will give you an excellent cardiovascular workout, and this is what we recommend that you ultimately aim for. If you are already very fit, we recommend that instead of performing the optional cardio routine, you simply put more effort, force, and intensity into each isometric exercise.

At the same time, aim to keep the rest time between those exercises as brief as possible. This approach will help you work towards performing each exercise with an Ultra-High Intensity Ultra-Short Burst™ effect, which will greatly improve your overall fitness level and boost your Base Metabolic Rate (BMR).

However, if you are not already fit, you may wish to begin by simply allowing each isometric exercise to deliver all the cardio you need as you gradually build up your fitness and endurance levels. This gradual approach ensures that you feel confident and reassured in your fitness journey. Eventually, you will increase your fitness level to a point where you can gradually reduce the rest time between each exercise to a minimum that works best for you.

Once you have learned how to fully engage the muscles during each exercise with sufficient force, and at the same time, you have learned how to breathe fully, deeply, and naturally throughout each exercise. At the same time, you should be keeping the rest time between exercises to a minimum because this combination will have an excellent and beneficial cardiovascular effect.

Dynamic Flexation™

Dynamic Flexation™ is a technique we devised to help ensure that we gained maximum benefit from the isometric portion of our exercise regimens. I will recap and briefly summarise the Dynamic Flexation™ technique as originally laid out in "The 70 Second Difference™" book.

We always recommend that everyone who performs any kind of resistance exercise practices some form of Dynamic Flexation™ before performing any exercise. This will help to ensure that all muscles, tendons, ligaments, joints, and your spine have become naturally and properly engaged in the correct biomechanical exercise position.

We would never recommend that you immediately apply maximum power and force as soon as you assume any exercise position. This is unless you are a very experienced athlete or unless you are training with a qualified coach to perform a certain type of isometric exercise to develop extra power, such as a static-dynamic or explosive/ballistic isometric technique. Instead, we recommend that you always breathe naturally as you gradually flex and engage your muscles and joints into performing the exercise.

To perform Dynamic Flexation™, you gradually flex your grip and the muscles you are about to exercise while applying an increasing level of force immediately before performing the exercise. The exercise is then performed, and to disengage from it, we recommend reversing the Dynamic Flexation™ engagement process.

We prefer to gradually apply tension and force to the exercise through Dynamic Flexation™, typically for between 2 and 3 seconds, or even for as long as 4 seconds if needed. This all takes place before beginning to count the required 7-second exercise time of the isometric contraction.

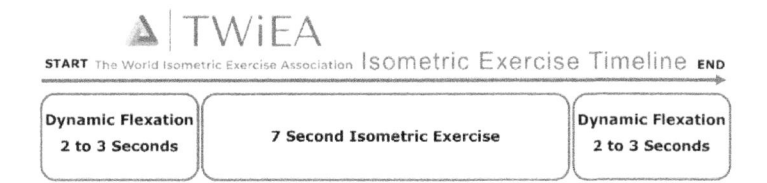

△ | TWiEA
START The World Isometric Exercise Association Isometric Exercise Timeline END

Dynamic Flexation 2 to 3 Seconds	7 Second Isometric Exercise	Dynamic Flexation 2 to 3 Seconds

We prefer using one deep, full breath in and out to count each second that has elapsed more accurately. This way, you will time each exercise more accurately and not be tempted to hold your breath at any point, which is a mistake that beginners often make.

Similarly, at the end of an exercise, we do not recommend that it be ended abruptly. Instead, we recommend reversing the Dynamic Flexation™ technique so that you gradually relax as you slightly move each muscle and joint out of the exercise position.

This process helps enormously because when you are in a good position, you will gain the maximum benefit from each exercise you perform.

Dynamic Flexation™ is when you move and adjust your feet, legs, hips, and especially your hands as you gradually assume a solid position and handgrip. As you flex and move, you will be making micro-adjustments.

All exercises will be performed best if you assume a correct and solid handgrip, fist clench, or foot position, etc. One of the most important aspects of assuming the correct exercise position begins with your grip.

Without a solid grip on a bar, handle, or anything else you need to hold while exercising, you will naturally be setting yourself up to perform sub-maximally. You can also be helping to develop injuries which can include sore elbows, joints, ligaments, and tendons.

Dynamic Flexation™ is a concept that embraces the broader principles of motor unit recruitment and "Henneman's Size Principle" to increase the contractile strength of a muscle.

Elwood Henneman's principle stated that under load, the motor units in a muscle are engaged according to their magnitude of force output, from the smallest to the largest, and in task-appropriate order.

This means that the slow-twitch, low-force, fatigue-resistant muscle fibres are activated before any fast-twitch, high-force muscle fibres are engaged, which are less fatigue-resistant. Since the body naturally works in this way, it enables precise and finely controlled force to be delivered at all levels of output.

This also means that fatigue will always be minimised when exercising or performing tasks in daily life. It will also be proportional to the sequential engagement of the most appropriate muscle fibres.

Isometric Exercises and Blood Pressure

Some exercise critics point out that performing an isometric exercise raises blood pressure. However, these people conveniently forget that the same is true of all other forms of exercise, including freehand callisthenics and traditional isotonic resistance training with weights.

ALL physical activity, especially exercise, will cause your blood pressure to rise for a short time. Providing that you are in good health, if you always breathe deeply, naturally and normally when performing any exercise, any rise in blood pressure will soon return to normal when the exercise stops. The faster this happens, the fitter you are.

For advanced athletes and/or those who have been used to hard and intense isometric training for a long time, you will already have made significant progress in strengthening your heart and circulatory system.

For those who are new to isometric training, just like with any form of exercise, the best way to get into it is by taking it slowly and less intensely at first. Newcomers to exercise, especially isometrics, should always focus on applying less force and breathing fully and deeply throughout all exercises. NEVER HOLD YOUR BREATH!

Under strict medical supervision, even those with Coronary Artery Disease and high blood pressure should be able to increase their physical activity levels with a reasonable degree of safety. However, if you already suffer from high blood pressure, you should always exercise at a much lower level of intensity than someone who has no physical issues.

FURTHERMORE, EVERYONE, ESPECIALLY PEOPLE WITH HYPERTENSION OR ANY FORM OF CARDIOVASCULAR DISEASE, SHOULD ALWAYS CHECK WITH THEIR DOCTOR BEFORE BEGINNING ANY KIND OF EXERCISE ROUTINE.

Rest and Recovery

Many factors must be considered when calculating your ideal recovery period. These include your age, current health and fitness level, the quantity of exercise you have done, and, most importantly, the intensity of the exercise.

Some people need a recovery period of between 24 and 48 hours; for others, it may be as brief as 12 to 24 hours. As a rule, the recovery period will always incrementally increase as the intensity of the exercises increases towards an individual's 100% potential maximum capacity. Always be aware of this, and make sure that you factor this into your rest and recovery time calculations. The diagram will help to outline this.

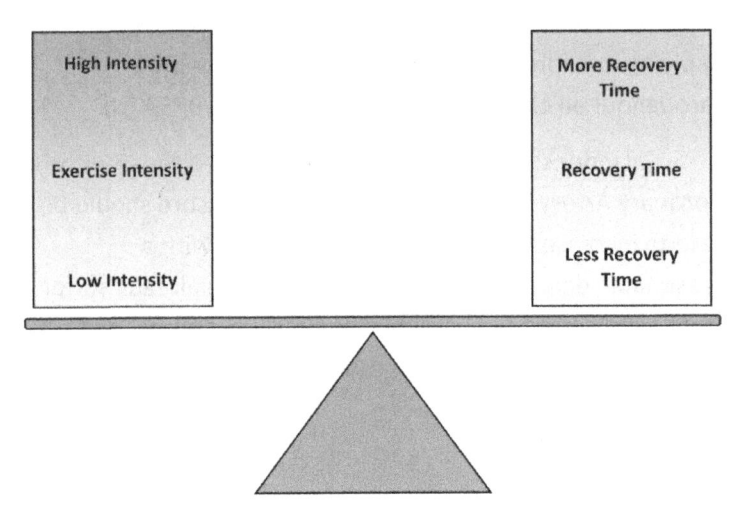

Sports scientist J. Atha's research revealed something remarkable. It showed that the average person could safely perform an exercise like this daily without overtraining when performing isometric contraction exercises at two-thirds of an individual's maximum capacity.

Standard isometric contraction exercises can be safely performed daily by almost anyone of almost any age and in almost any physical condition as a means of strength development, body shaping, and even bodybuilding.

However, we recommend a full rest day between sessions for more intense workouts due to the higher demands placed upon the central nervous system (CNS) and the time needed to recover and fully benefit from the exercise.

Several other factors affect post-exercise recovery. These include a balanced and properly executed stretching routine and getting enough quality sleep. While you sleep, your body releases certain hormones that help you repair and rebuild damaged tissue and that will directly help your muscles grow.

Adequate Nutrition is Vital

Quality post-exercise nutrition will help your body repair itself faster, decrease your recovery time, and maximise the benefits gained from the exercise. Research shows that post-exercise immunodepression peaks if you exercise longer than you are currently capable, and problems are enhanced due to reduced or inadequate nutrition.

Hydration is also one of the most important factors in your recovery and for your overall health, especially since your muscles are mostly composed of water.

Early studies suggested a 30 to 60-minute window after exercise when you need to eat, after which your body begins to draw upon itself to repair and recover from your workout. Later studies found that this window can be anything from 1 to 3 hours depending on the workout type, applied force, overall intensity, and goals. On average, since most leave 60 minutes after food before hard exercise, and if a workout lasts an average of 45 minutes, then a 30 to 45-minute window to eat after exercise will mean it has been up to 150 minutes (2.5 hours) since your last food; therefore, the earlier suggested 30–45-minute window still makes sense for most people especially if they want to build more muscle and strength.

Most people mistakenly consume excessive amounts of protein at the expense of other key nutrients, such as carbohydrates. Therefore, in doing this, they are working against their best interests and overall optimum health. One of the key nutrients that have been found to help enormously when in recovery from prolonged periods of heavy exercise is carbohydrates. A lot of research supports the hypothesis that carbohydrate is the most important nutritional factor in preventing post-exercise immunodepression.

Most do not realise that the protein composition of human muscle is typically only somewhere in the region of between 18/9% and 21% protein (average 20%), and the rest is made up of water, glucose, lipids, and carbohydrates, etc. We will not go into more detail here; however, if you want to learn more about this and many other surprising nuggets of useful information about sensible nutrition and exercise, then they can be found in The 70 Second Difference book.

Strength, Stamina, Endurance, and Resilience

Understanding the difference between strength, stamina, and endurance is important because once you do, you will be able to devise the most suitable workout routines for your body type.

Muscular strength is possibly best understood as a muscle's capacity to exert force against resistance or weight. This is comparatively easy to measure because one's ability to lift a given amount of weight for a single repetition is a good measure of strength.

Stamina is the length of time at which a muscle or group of muscles can perform at or near its maximum capacity. For example, the number of squats you can perform with a given weight that is 90% of your maximum would be a measure of your stamina or the distance that you can carry a similarly heavy object such as an anvil.

Endurance is all about time and your ability to perform a certain muscular action for a prolonged period, regardless of the capacity at which you are working.

Resilience is all about your ability to recover from whatever stresses and demands are placed on your muscles. However, resilience is mostly all about your state of mind, your mental toughness and ability to endure, perform and deliver under pressure, and how you recover quickly emotionally.

Your body's muscular composition will always determine your performance in certain sports. The amount of slow-twitch muscle fibres you possess will determine your performance at endurance-related events, and both type A and type B fast-twitch muscle fibres are all about explosive power and your ability to maintain it.

In simple terms, if you possess mostly slow-twitch muscle fibres, you will naturally be better suited to endurance sports. Alternatively, you are a natural weightlifter if you possess mostly fast-twitch muscle fibres.

It is important to note that no matter what your natural predisposition might be in this respect, with the correct training regimen, it is still possible to significantly increase your abilities in your naturally weaker opposing areas of speciality.

Chapter 3:
Proprietary Isometric Exercise Equipment

We highly recommend and endorse the Iso-Bow®. as an exercise tool. This inexpensive little device is amazingly versatile and allows self-resisted isometric, isotonic, and functional isokinetic exercises to be performed easily. The Iso-Bow® provides the user with a biomechanically sound grip handle, which allows almost all exercises to be performed more effectively and with greater ease and comfort.

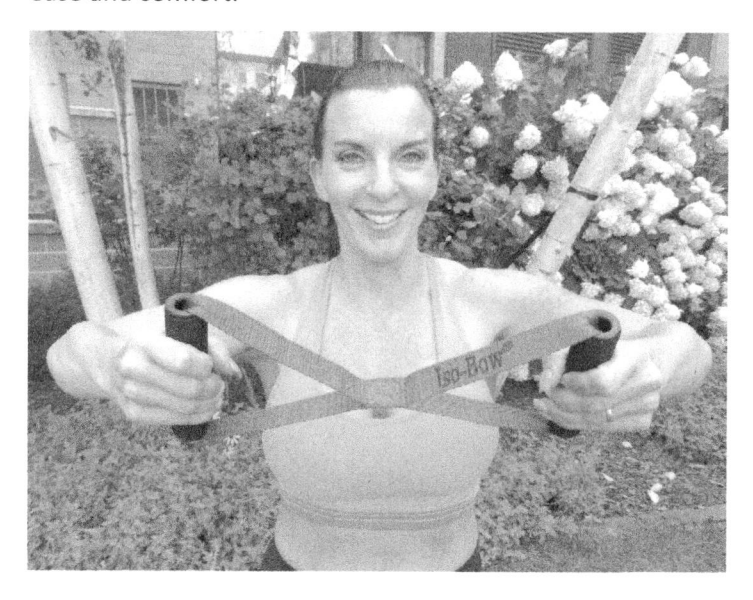

With a pair of Iso-Bows®, you can effectively exercise every major muscle group of the body and even perform advanced exercises such as pull-ups, the isometric squat, and the isometric deadlift. The level of workout you can get from using a pair of Iso-Bows® can range from an easy low-level beginner's workout right up to a very high-intensity professional athlete level of workout. Amazingly, you can do all of this without any adjustment being needed to the Iso-Bows®. Each user will benefit proportionately, according to the amount of effort, force, and intensity that is applied during each exercise.

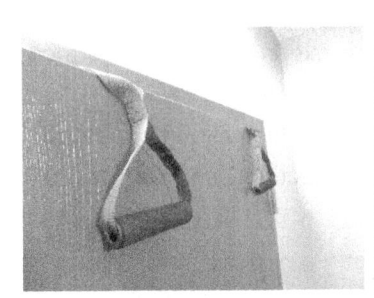

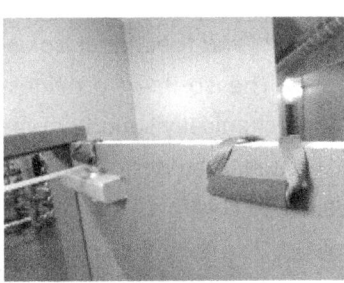

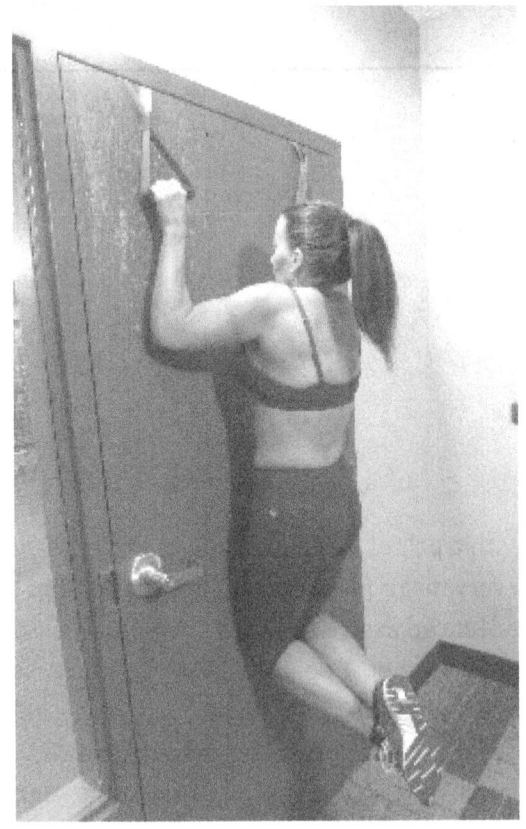

One of the standout features of the Iso-Bow® is its portability. It's so compact that it can easily fit into your pocket, handbag, briefcase, or backpack. This means you can take your workout with you wherever you go, making it the perfect companion for your busy lifestyle.

Perhaps the best-known of all isometric/isotonic home exercise devices is the Bullworker®, which has been a best-seller since its launch in the early 1960s. Today, it is still a best-selling device, and with good reason: It works. The smaller "partner" device is called the Steel Bow®, and both have interchangeable springs so that men and women of all strength levels and abilities can use them with roughly equal effectiveness.

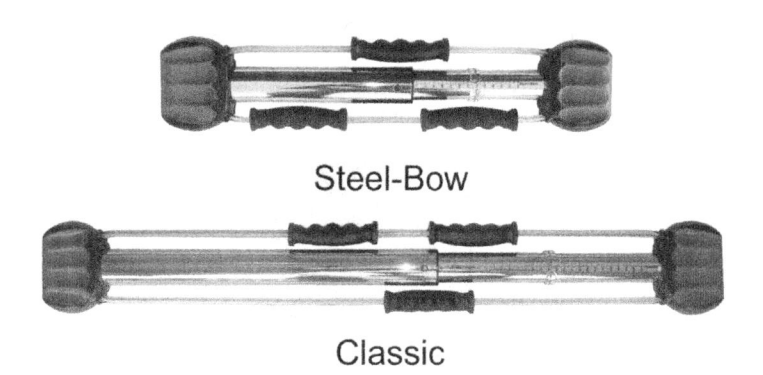

Steel-Bow

Classic

Securing the Iso-Bow® With Your Feet

When performing leg exercises such as squats and lunges, as well as lower back and glute exercises such as the deadlift, it becomes necessary to secure the Iso-Bow® using your feet properly. There are several ways in which the Iso-Bow® can be secured using your feet, and your preference of how you do this will depend upon many factors, such as your foot size, choice of footwear, and ease of operation.

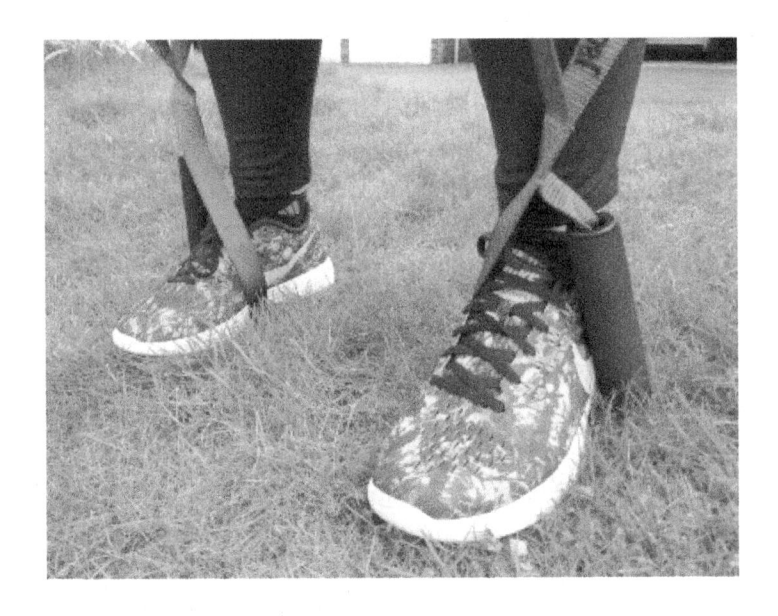

You can secure the Iso-Bow® with your foot inside one of the handles. To do this, adjust the handgrip to one side, usually the foot's outer side, and then place your feet inside the loop like a stirrup.

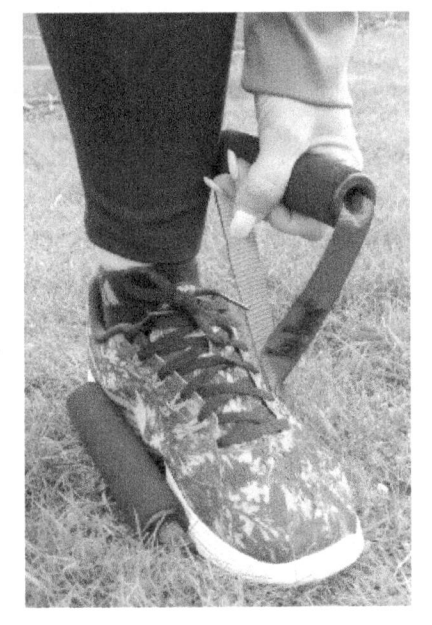

Another method is to place the Iso-Bow® flat on the floor and then stand on one side of the straps so that the handle of the same side sits flush with your inner foot. In this position, your bodyweight combined with the handle pressing against the inner side of your foot enables you to pull safely and securely.

The final method is to simply place each foot through one end of an Iso-Bow®, stepping onto the foam hand grip as you do so. This method is slightly less stable than the other two methods.

However, if the foot can be pushed far enough through the loop of the Iso-Bow® handle, then the handle will slightly raise the level of your heel, making it easier for some people to squat or lunge.

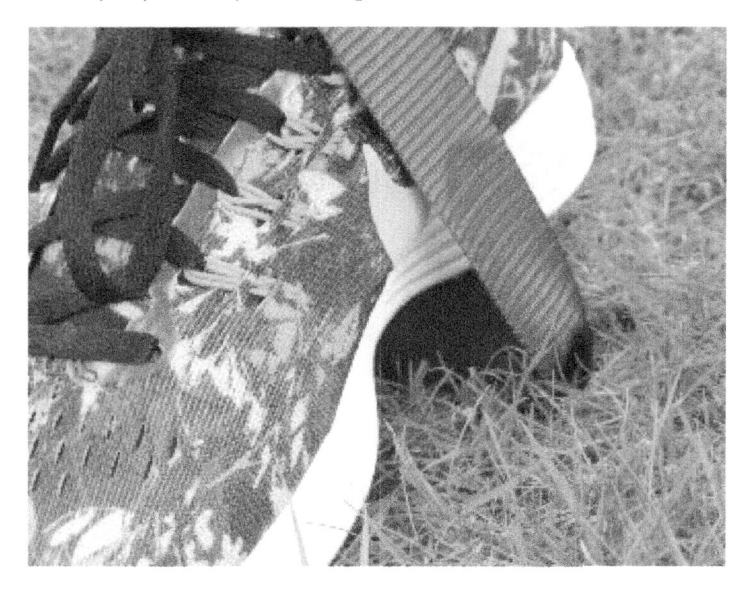

Naturally, safety is always a top priority, so whichever method you ultimately choose to use, you should always make sure that when securing the Iso-Bow® with your feet, there is never any chance of it slipping while you exercise.

Chapter 4: About the Exercise Model

Helen Renée is an American who is married to a Brit. She was born in Minnesota and grew up in Northern Alaska after her father became an Ice Road Trucker.

Helen went from being 40 lbs overweight to a contest-winning condition almost effortlessly in less than 6 months, with workout sessions lasting no longer than 10 minutes daily.

Helen is an isometric exercise expert instructor and champion Bikini Fitness Athlete who achieved spectacular contest-winning results after meeting her exercise scientist husband.

Helen's husband is one of the world's leading experts on isometric exercise plant-based nutrition and was a former coach to the 4-times World's Strongest Man, Jon Pall Sigmarsson of Iceland.

Currently, Helen has co-authored 21 fitness books, and since she and her husband share a common fascination with mysteries and the paranormal, they have co-authored a best-selling book on the subject.

Since meeting and marrying her British husband, they have enjoyed a joyous journey together, discovering the many differences between the two countries, which share a common language and culture.

They began writing down these stories and anecdotes and very soon had enough to produce a fun-filled and light-hearted book about what it is like to Be American Married to a Brit.

Helen is remarkably strong with the exceptional power-to-weight ratio one would expect from a former gymnast. She is also an isometric and TRISOmetric™ exercise instructor, consultant, and instructor-trainer for TWiEA™, The World Isometric Exercise Association. www.TWiEA.com – www.HelenRenee.com

The following pictures are of Helen Renée taken in January 2015 before she started performing a daily 10 x 7-second total-body exercise isometric exercise routine.

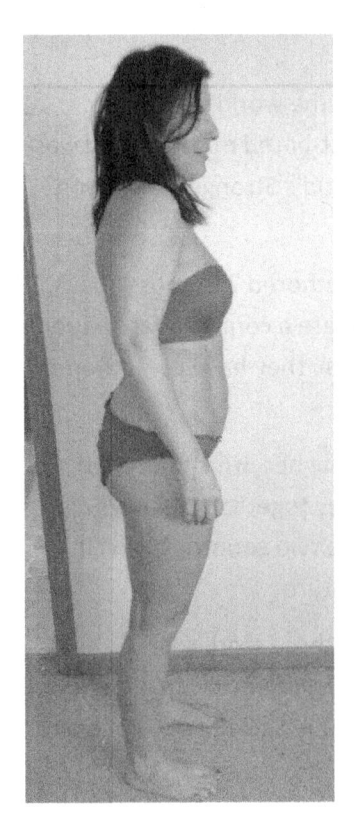

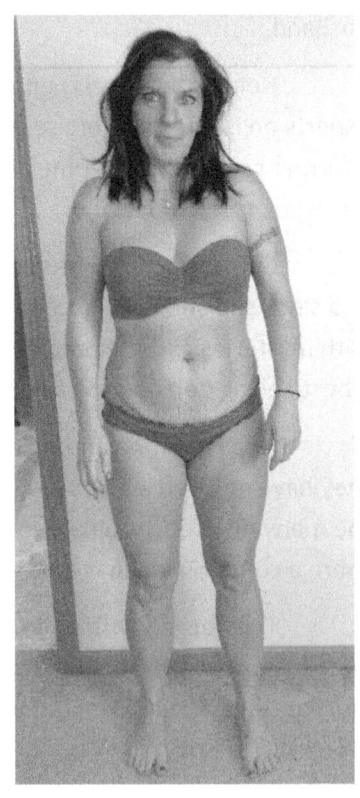

The following pictures on the next pages are of Helen Renée exactly one year later, in January 2016. She became a contest-winning Bikini Fitness competitor performing nothing more than daily isometric exercise training lasting only minutes each day. Now, Helen trains using only isometric exercises because they are so effective. She exercises regularly each day and applies more force to each exercise than a normal person who simply wants to get a little stronger and fitter and maintain a good overall body shape. Helen also eats sensibly.

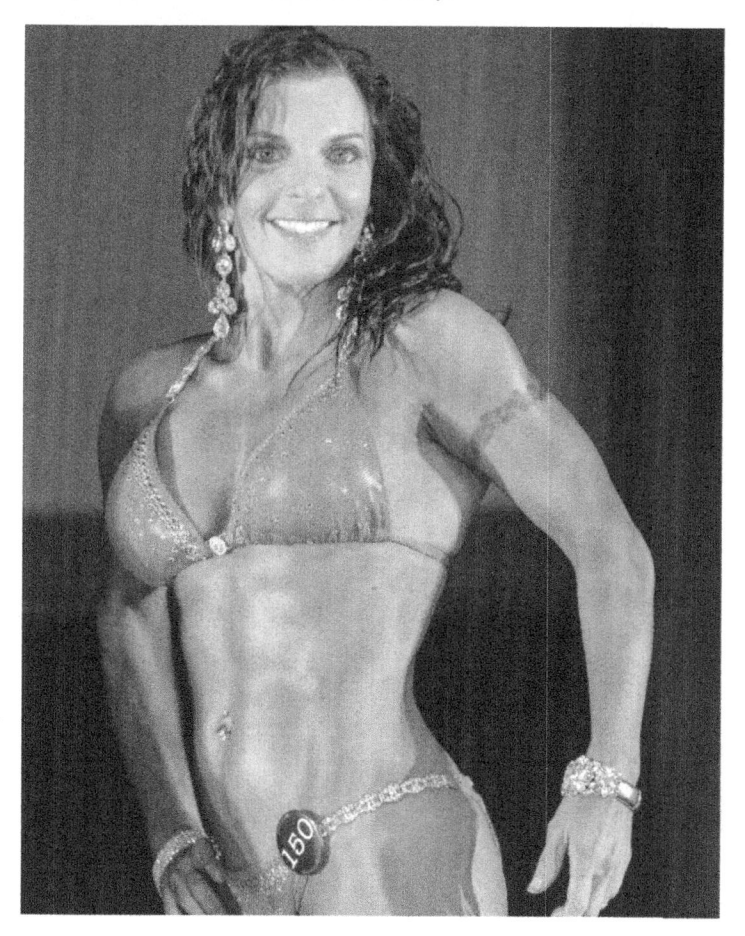

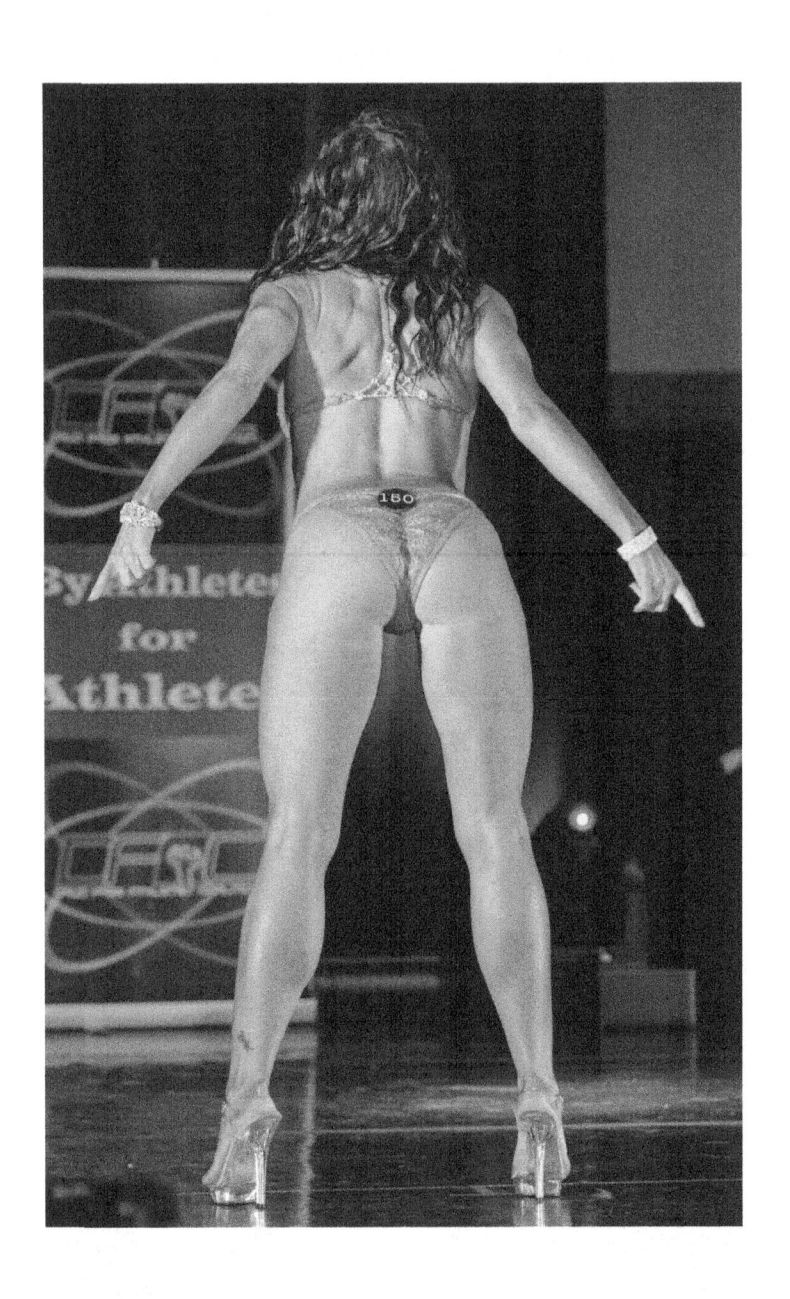

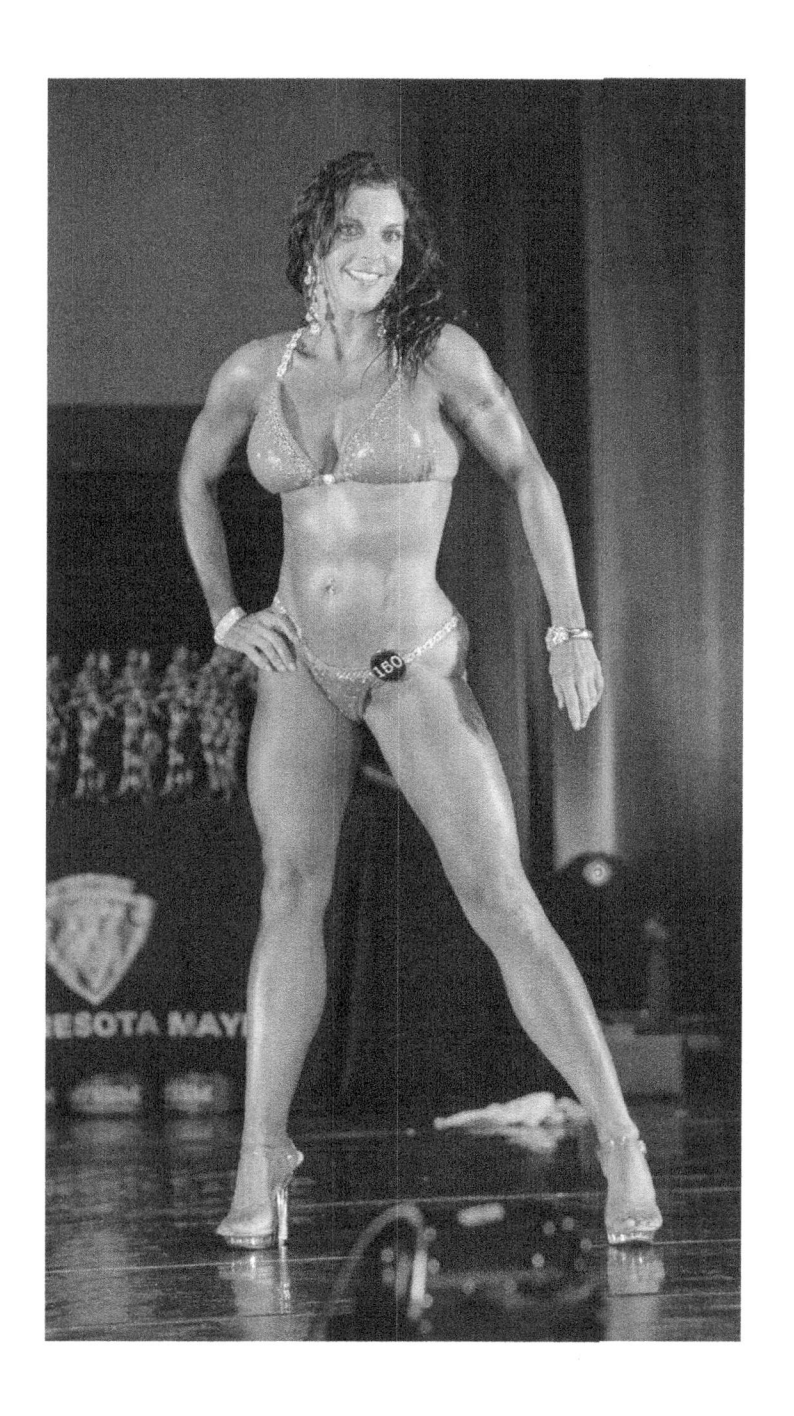

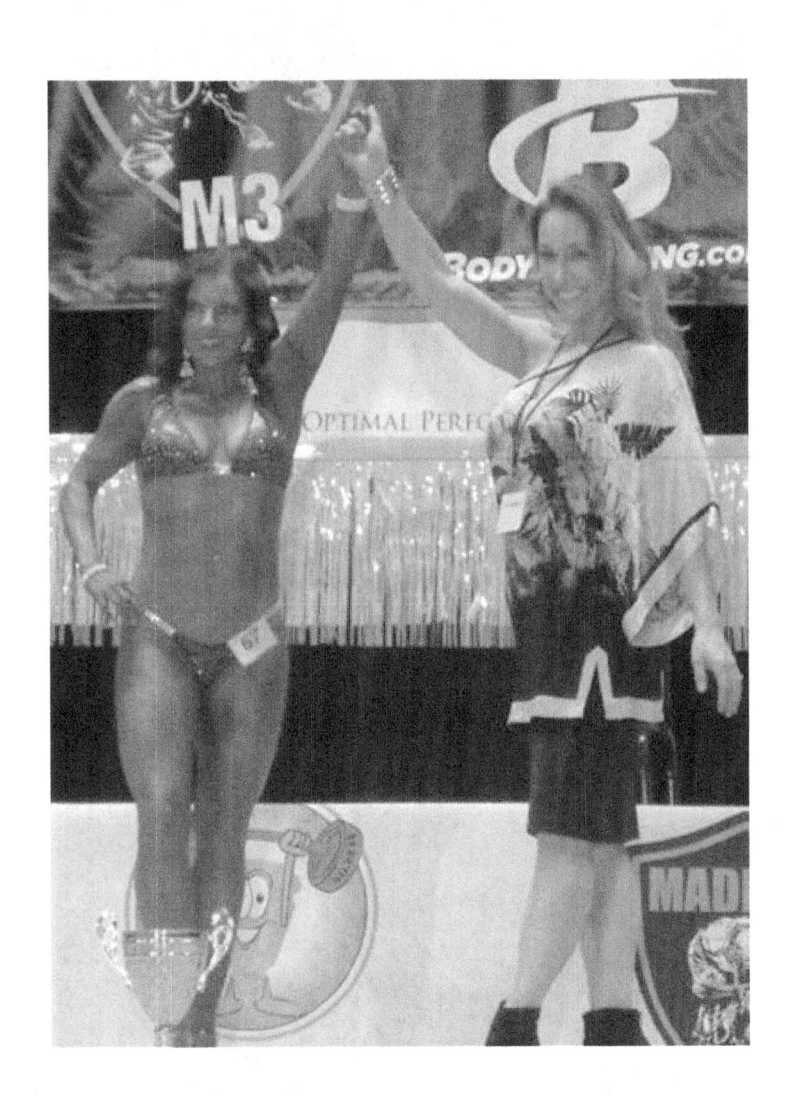

The Author and an Isometric Experiment

The following picture is of my arm, taken in December 2016. It is the result of a year-long experiment to see what results could be gained through a basic high-intensity isometric exercise routine using only the minimum number of exercises.

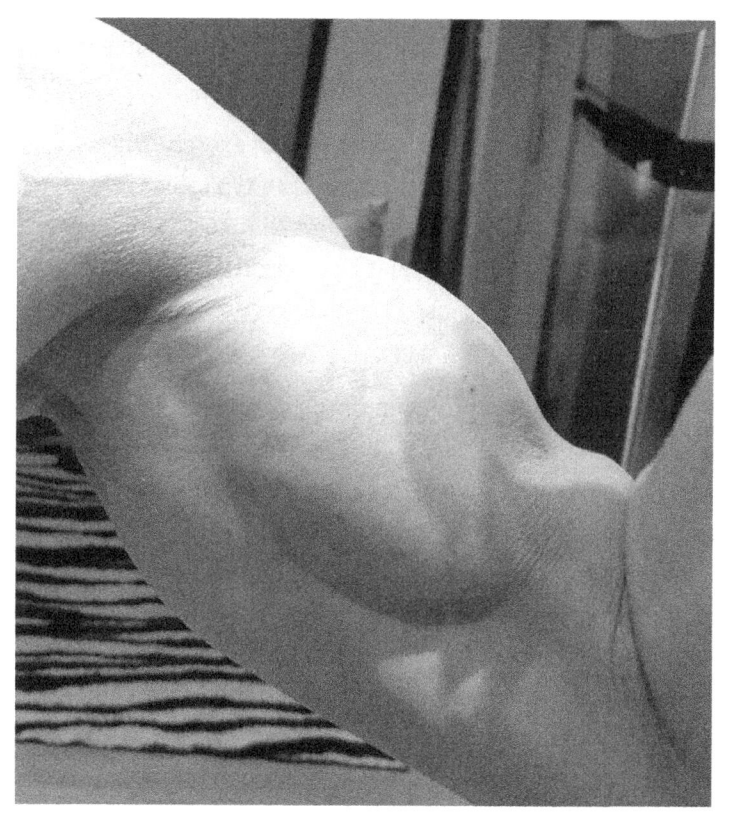

My arm after 1 year of basic isometric maintenance training. This picture was taken to record the results of the experiment in December 2016.

The routine allowed just 1 x 7-second isometric exercise per muscle/muscle group per day at a target level of applied force/intensity of between 75% and 80%.

For one year, starting in January 2016, I performed a daily 10-exercise x 7-second total-body isometric routine. It is common for even the most experienced athletes to count the elapsed exercise time increasingly quickly, almost in direct proportion to an increasing level of applied force/intensity. Therefore, I typically aimed to perform a 10-second isometric hold for each exercise, and this way, I would always reach the desired goal of 7 seconds in good style.

My target level of force for each exercise was around 75-80%, slightly higher than the typically recommended average of two-thirds or 66.6%. However, this still effectively meant that I exercised each of my biceps for a total of between just 21 and 30 seconds per week, nothing more.

Amazingly, at the end of the year-long experiment, I achieved an improvement in both the strength and size of each arm, albeit slightly. Even though I am well-versed in the science of isometrics I still found it remarkable because it was in exchange for a maximum of 30 seconds per week of exercise time. Once again, this only reinforced that the best results are always gained through pinpoint focus, high intensity, and never confusing activity with accomplishment.

Chapter 5:
Things to Remember Before You Begin

- The first and perhaps the most important thing to remember is: **NEVER HOLD YOUR BREATH AT ANY TIME.**
- Breathing in and out naturally during all isometric exercises will also help you count the number of elapsed seconds much more accurately, with one full breath in and out taking approximately one second.
- We recommend that you read the instructions about each exercise carefully.
- Always leave a safe distance between you and others if exercising with any proprietary device or IIED (Improvised Isometric Exercise Device)
- Always check the structural integrity of any type of exercise device. If there is any doubt about the structural integrity, then do not use it for exercise or any other purpose.
- Before use, double-check that all adjustable joints on the exercise device and/or IIED are secure.
- Weight loss/fat loss will ONLY occur when any exercise plan is used in conjunction with a calorie-controlled diet.
- It is critically important to completely focus your mind on the exercise being performed. Envision the muscle you are exercising growing larger and stronger.
- Always consult a professional coach to devise a detailed stretching routine, this will ensure that you

are stretching the areas effectively rather than risking injury.
- ⚠ Always ensure that a stable line of biomechanical progression is achieved before engaging in and performing any exercise.
- ⚠ Warming-up, stretching, and cooling down are three of the most overlooked yet essential elements of exercise, and we cannot stress their importance strongly enough.
- ⚠ During ANY form of physical exercise, including isometrics, if you apply too much force too soon, then you may inadvertently strain a muscle. Isometric exercise is particularly intense, and a single isometric exercise engages many more muscle fibres than even high-intensity weight training and at a much higher level.

For safety's sake, we always recommend using Dynamic Flexation™ to gradually and progressively engage your muscles in ANY exercise, especially isometrics, according to what we call The ISOfitness Exercise Engagement Timeline™.

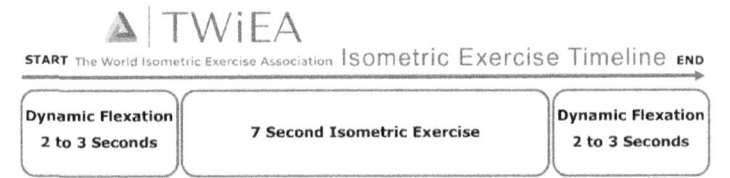

⚠ | TWiEA

START The World Isometric Exercise Association Isometric Exercise Timeline END

Dynamic Flexation 2 to 3 Seconds	7 Second Isometric Exercise	Dynamic Flexation 2 to 3 Seconds

The main benefit of properly warming up for several minutes before a workout is injury prevention and increasing your heart rate and circulation to your muscles, ligaments, and tendons. It is important to remember that warming-up and stretching are two different concepts and that stretching is not a good warm-up. This is because stretching will put the muscle in an un-contracted position and weaken it. Stretching is always best performed after a workout has been completed, together with a proper cool-down.

In addition to properly warming-up, always perform a gentle flex and stretch of the muscles and joints that are about to be exercised. For example, squatting down fully to flex the thighs and loosen the knees is always a good idea before performing any leg exercises. Dynamic Flexation™ performed before any exercise should help to ensure greater flexibility and increased blood supply to the muscles and surrounding tissue.

Isometric exercises are deceptively powerful. Even when engaging in what may feel like only moderate-intensity exercise, you are probably still engaging and contracting many more muscle fibres than you would in a similar isotonic exercise. Therefore, if you are in any doubt whatsoever, always perform the exercise with less force.

All exercises and workout plans work equally well for men and women. Both sexes can build strength, muscle, body build, or simply get into great shape if so desired, each according to their natural ability.

In our exercise resource books, the exercises listed are suggestions of what can be performed for each body part/muscle group. We are not suggesting that they should all be performed. Instead, users may wish to select the most suitable exercises from each section. In our course books, please perform the exercises according to the workout session notes.

Finally, please reread and review the 'Important General Safety and Health Guidelines' section to ensure that you have fully complied with all recommendations. Only start using the isometric or any exercise system with the full approval of your physician.

Chapter 6: Exercise Resources
Stomach Muscles - Club Pushdown

Stand upright with your feet approximately shoulder-width apart to perform the stomach muscles club pushdown. Hold the club upright on the ground or solid surface in front of you so that your elbows are slightly bent. Keep your arms locked so they do not move during the exercise. In this position, you should press the club down directly into the ground. You do this by bending slightly at the waist to engage and use your stomach muscles to push the club down. The harder you press and engage the stomach muscles, the more intense the exercise becomes, so be sure to exercise at a level of applied force that best suits you and your ability.

When you perform an isometric exercise, never hold your breath. Always breathe deeply and naturally, which will be about 10 full breaths in and out at a rate of about 1 second per full breath. Perform each exercise for no less than 7 seconds and no longer than 10.

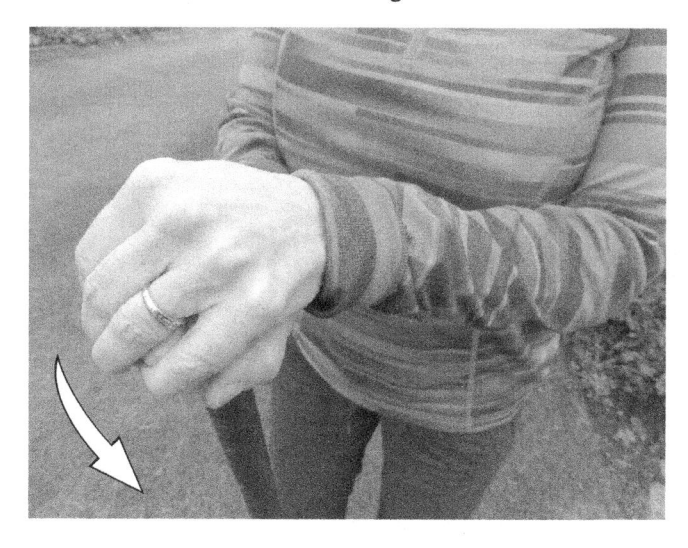

87

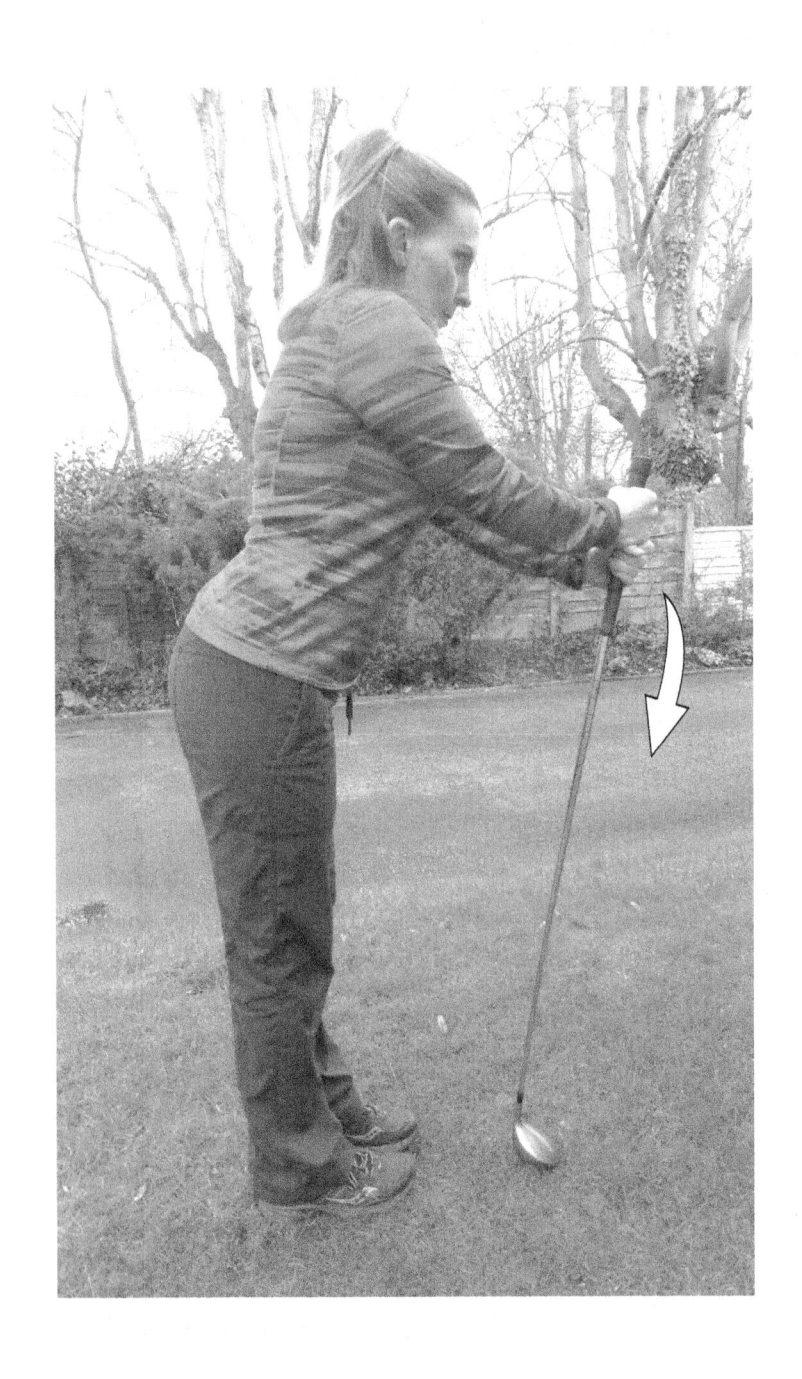

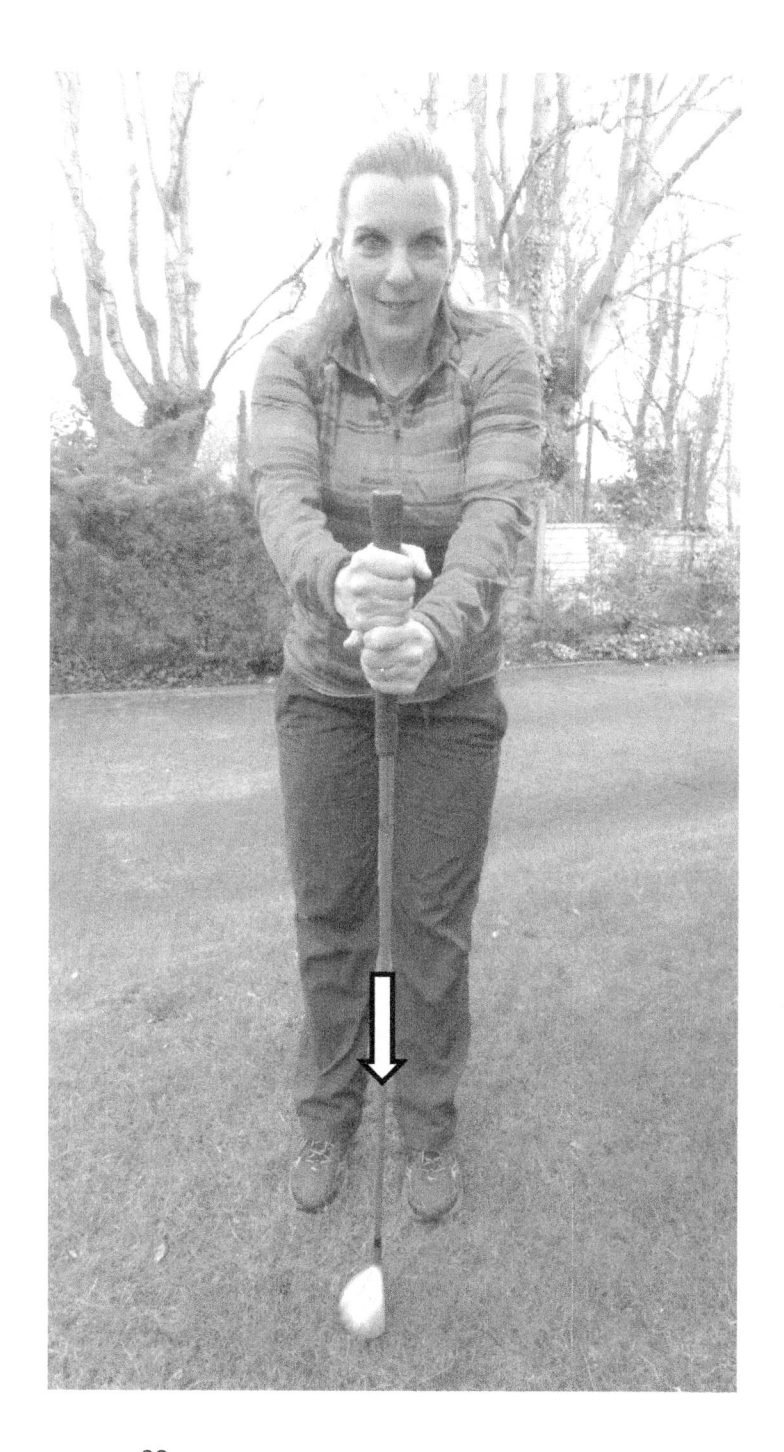

89

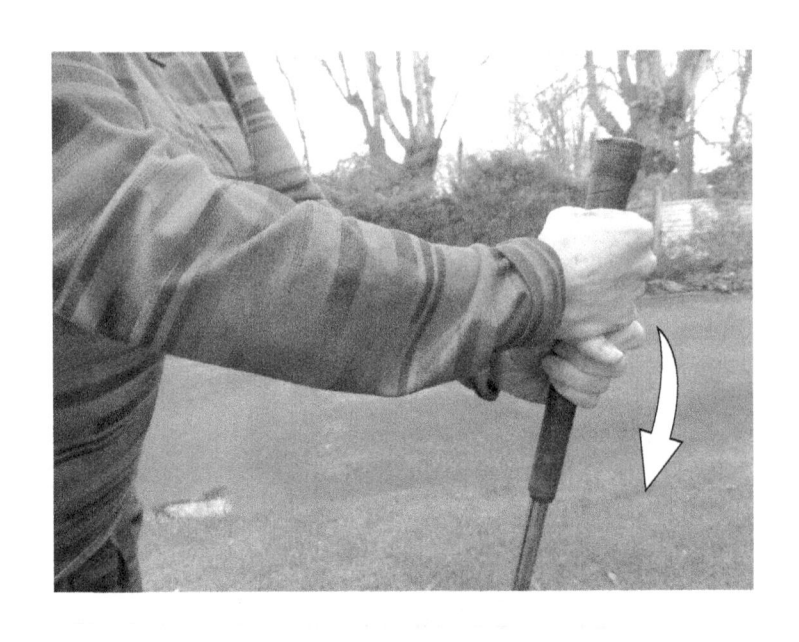

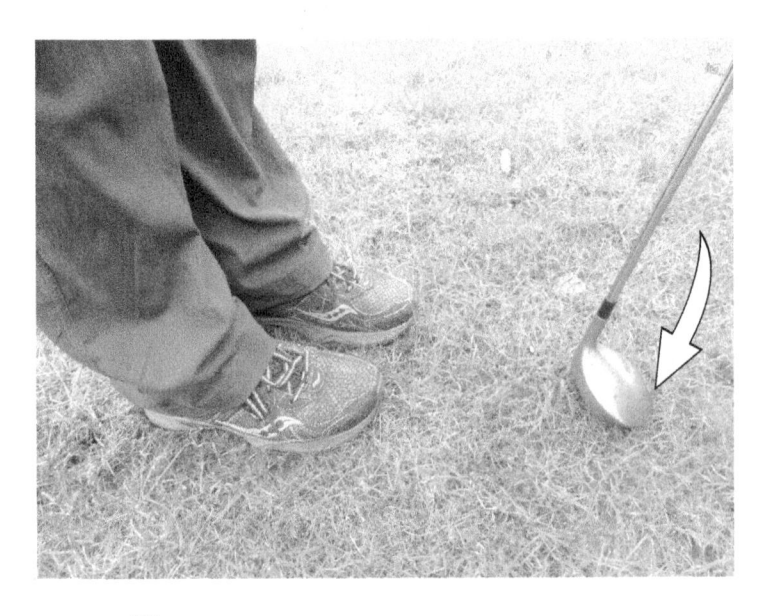

Stomach Muscles - Club Oblique Pushdown

Stand upright with your feet approximately shoulder-width apart to perform the stomach muscles club oblique pushdown. Hold the club upright on the ground or a solid surface to one side of you so that your elbows are slightly bent. Keep your arms locked so they do not move during the exercise. In this position, you should press the club down and slightly backwards into the ground. You do this by bending slightly at the waist to the same side as the club to engage and use your oblique stomach muscles to push the club down. The harder you press and engage the stomach muscles, the more intense the exercise becomes, so be sure to exercise at a level of applied force that best suits your ability. Be sure to exercise both sides of the body.

When you perform an isometric exercise, never hold your breath. Always breathe deeply and naturally, which will be about 10 full breaths in and out at a rate of about 1 second per full breath. Perform each exercise for no less than 7 seconds and no longer than 10.

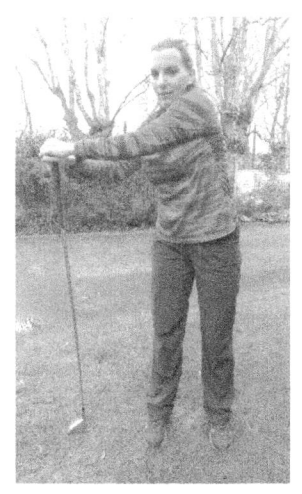

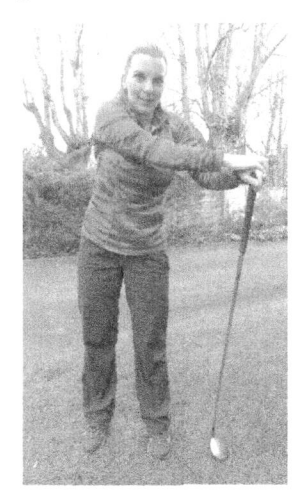

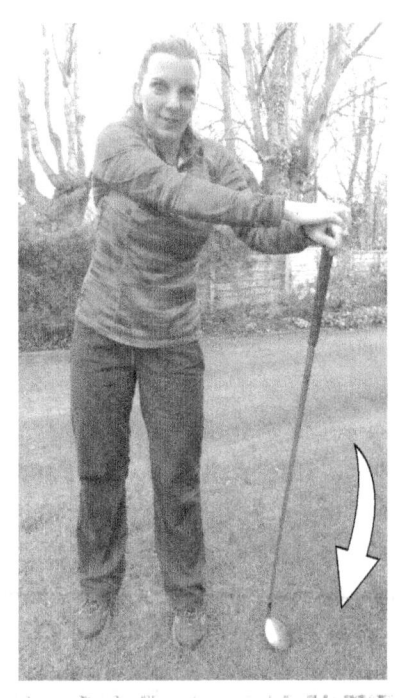

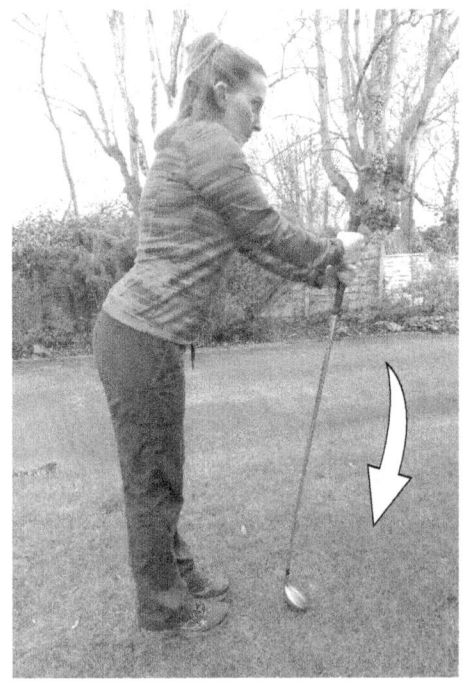

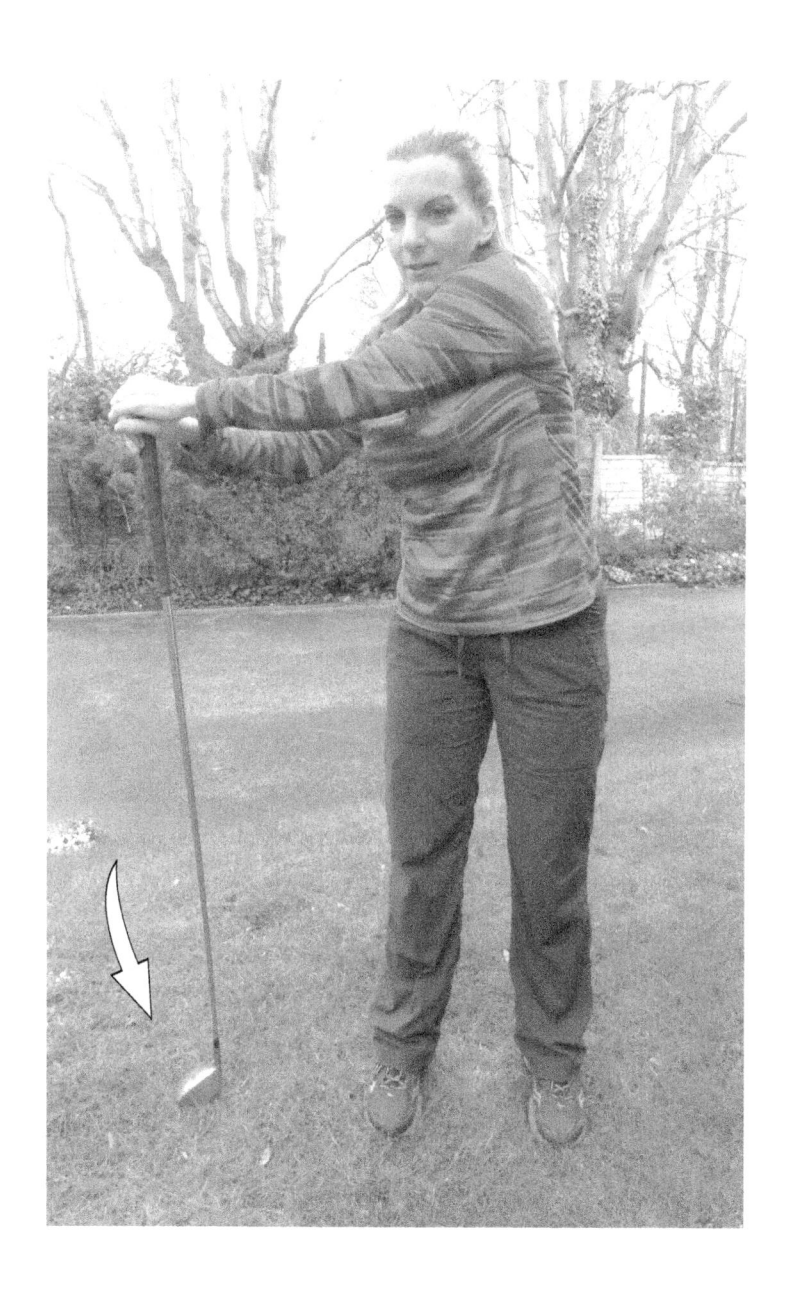

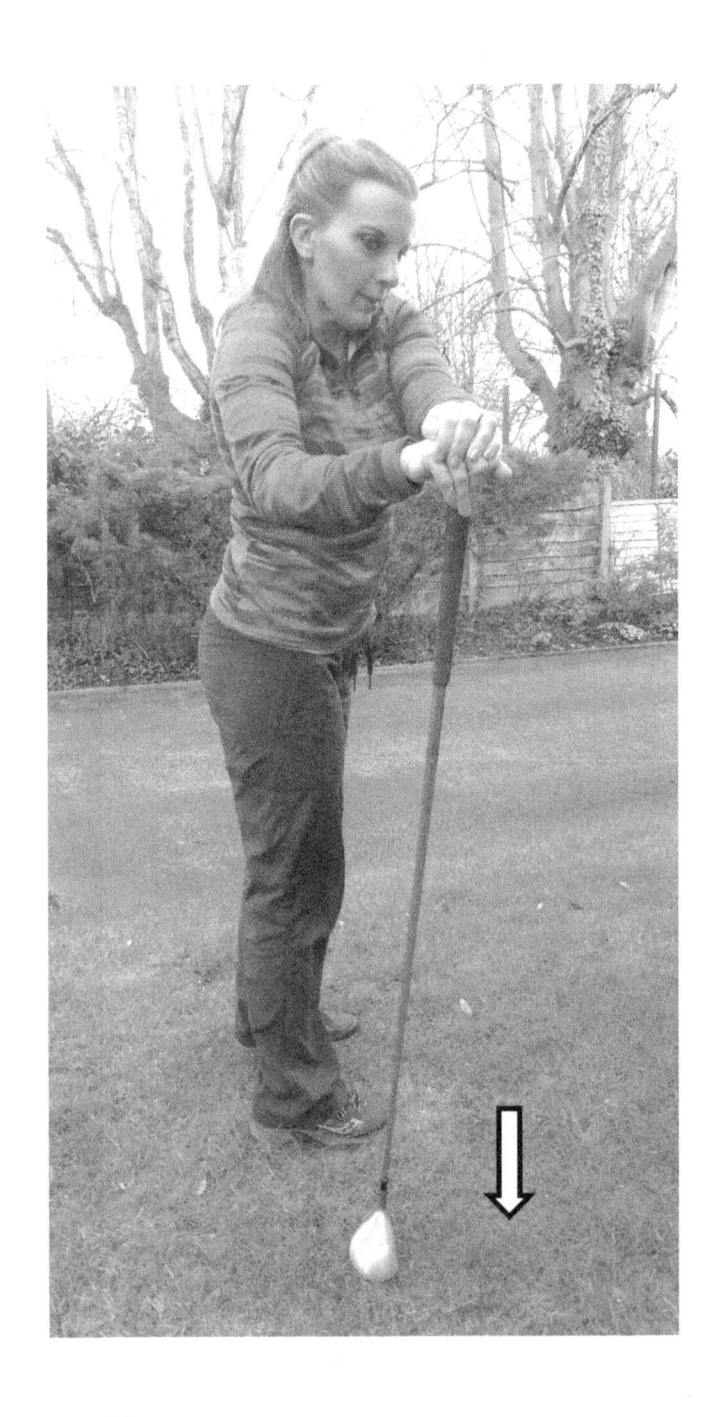

Arms – Upper Arm Club Under-Thigh Biceps Curl

To perform the upper arm club under-thigh curl, stand upright with your back against a solid object such as a rock, a tree, a wall, or a fence, etc. Raise one leg in front of you with the knee bent. Slide the club under that leg close to the bend in your knee. Hold the club in both hands about shoulder-width apart with your palms facing up. In this position, bend the arms in a curling motion until you reach the mid-point or maximum position you can attain. Even though you cannot raise the club any further, continue to try to do so and maintain a steady level of force to exercise the front upper arms. Press downward with your bent raised leg to apply even more force to the arms during this exercise if necessary. The harder you press and engage the biceps muscles, the more intense the exercise becomes. Be sure to exercise at a level of applied force and overall intensity that best suits your ability.

When you perform an isometric exercise, never hold your breath. Always breathe deeply and naturally, which will be about 10 full breaths in and out at a rate of about 1 second per full breath. Perform each exercise for no less than 7 seconds and no longer than 10.

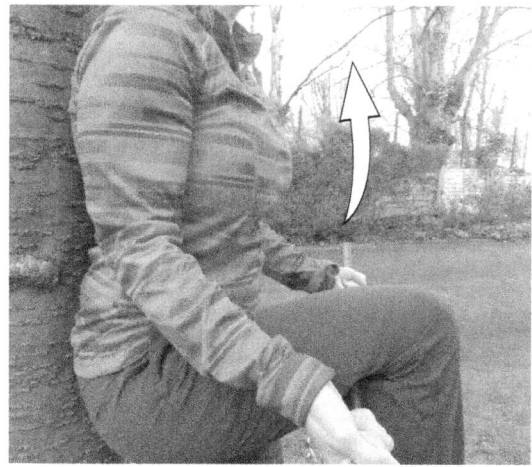

95

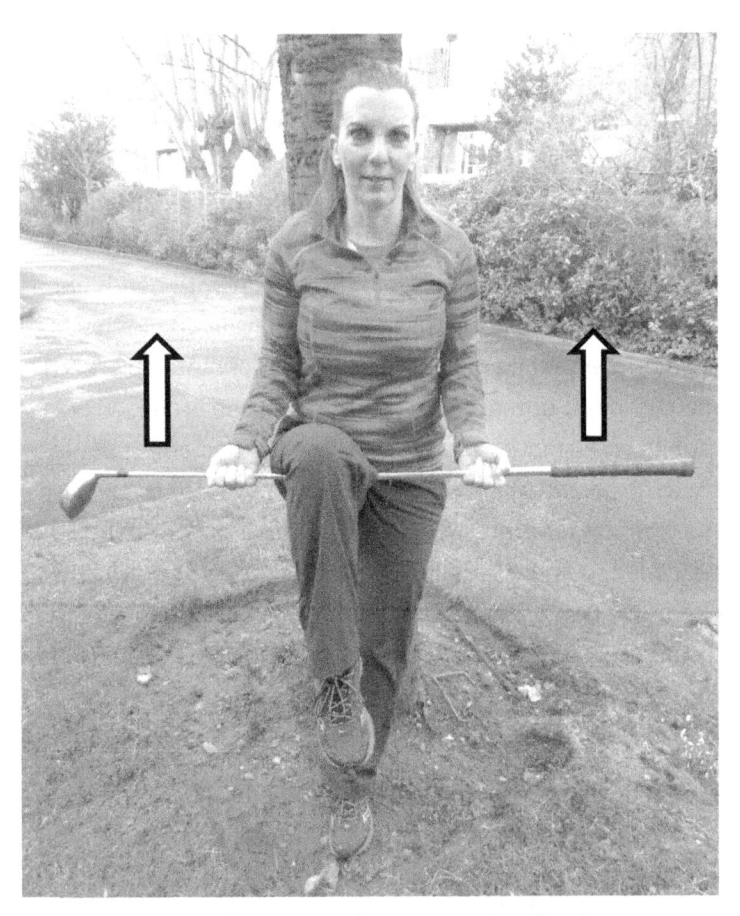

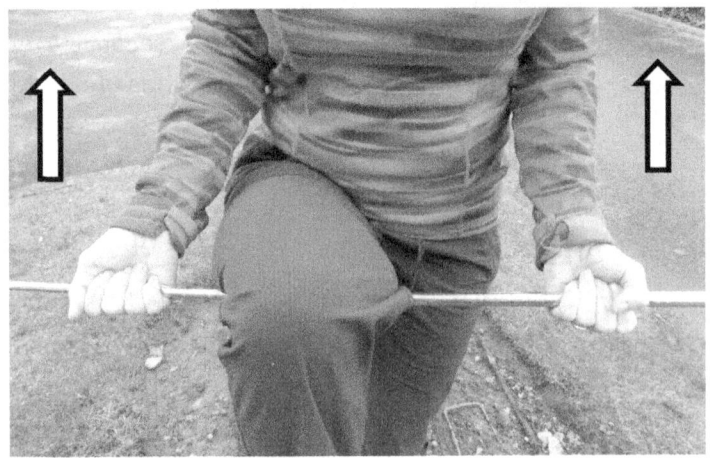

Arms – Upper Arm Triceps-Biceps

The Upper arm triceps-biceps exercise engages both the front and rear upper arms. The exercise is in two parts. One part exercises the front upper arm of one side of the body and simultaneously the rear upper arm of the other side. In simple terms, one arm/hand is attempting to raise, and the other arm/hand is pushing down Then, after a change of either grip position or direction of effort, the emphasis of the exercise reverses. Always be sure to exercise both arms/sides of the body equally in both directions. Be sure to keep the arms roughly bent at the midpoint with your elbows close to the body during the exercise. The harder you press and engage both the biceps and triceps muscles, the more intense the exercise becomes. Be sure to grip firmly and exercise at a force and overall intensity level that best suits your ability.

When you perform an isometric exercise, never hold your breath. Always breathe deeply and naturally, which will be about 10 full breaths in and out at a rate of about 1 second per full breath. Perform each exercise for no less than 7 seconds and no longer than 10.

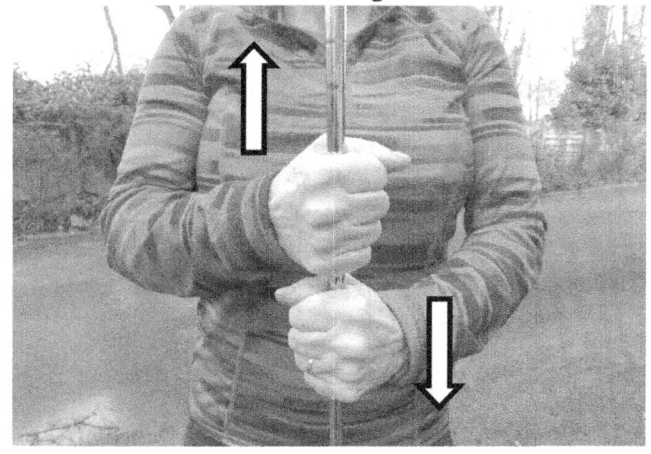

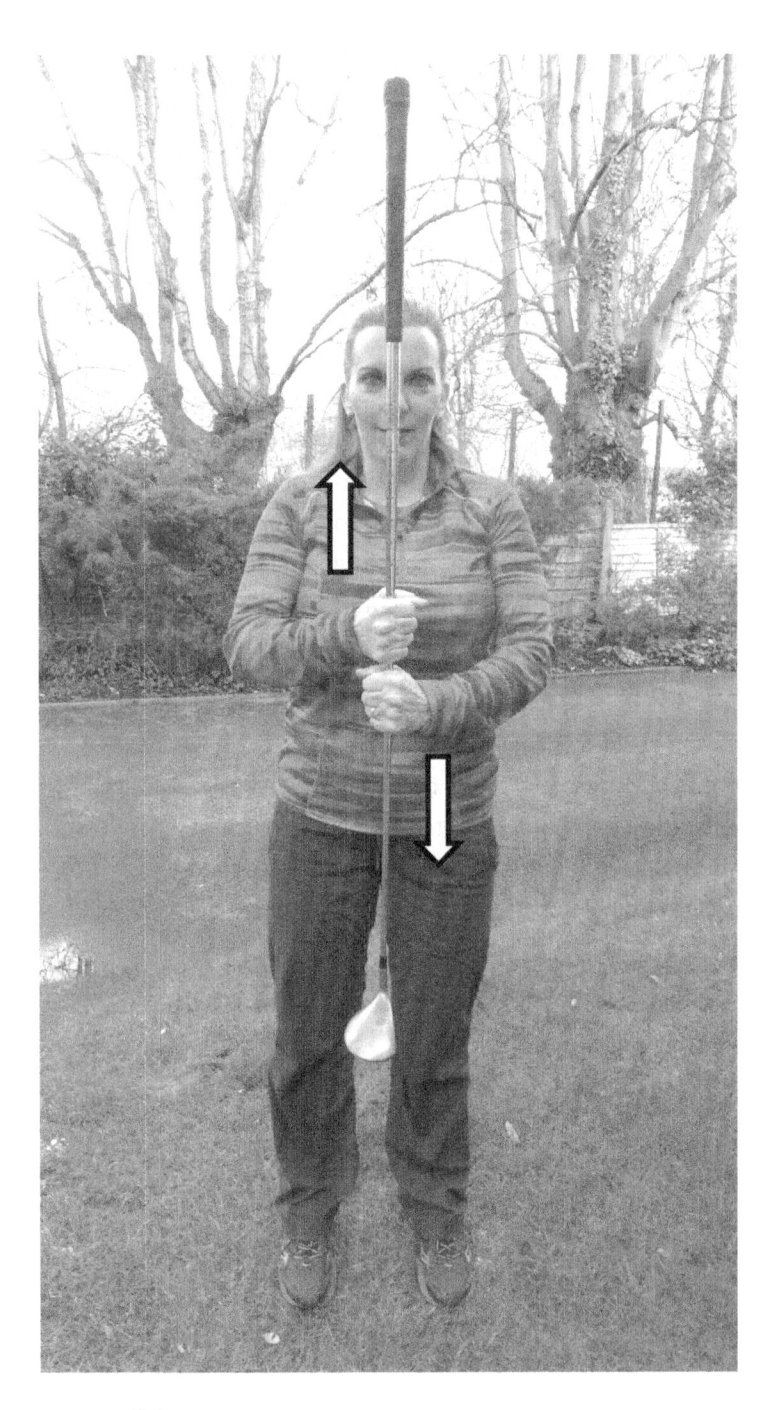

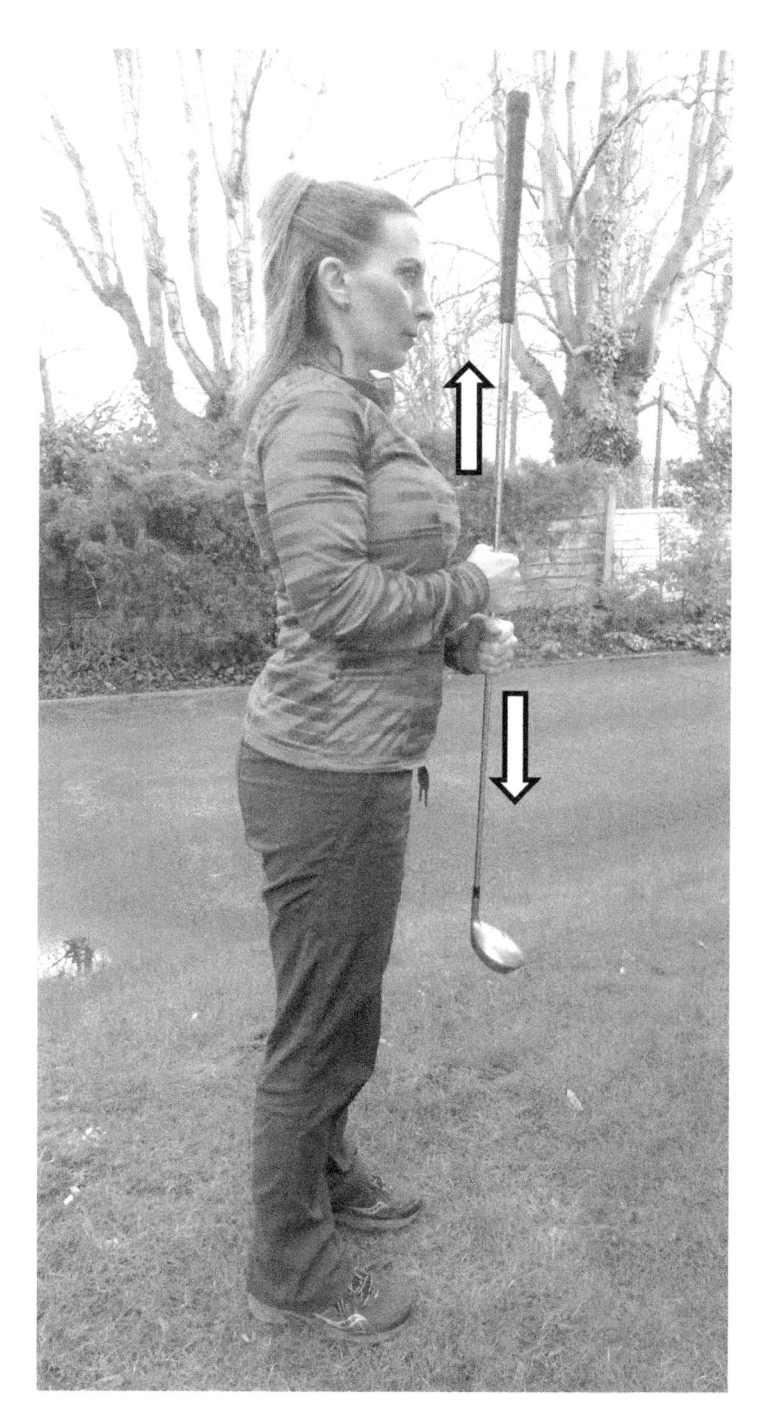

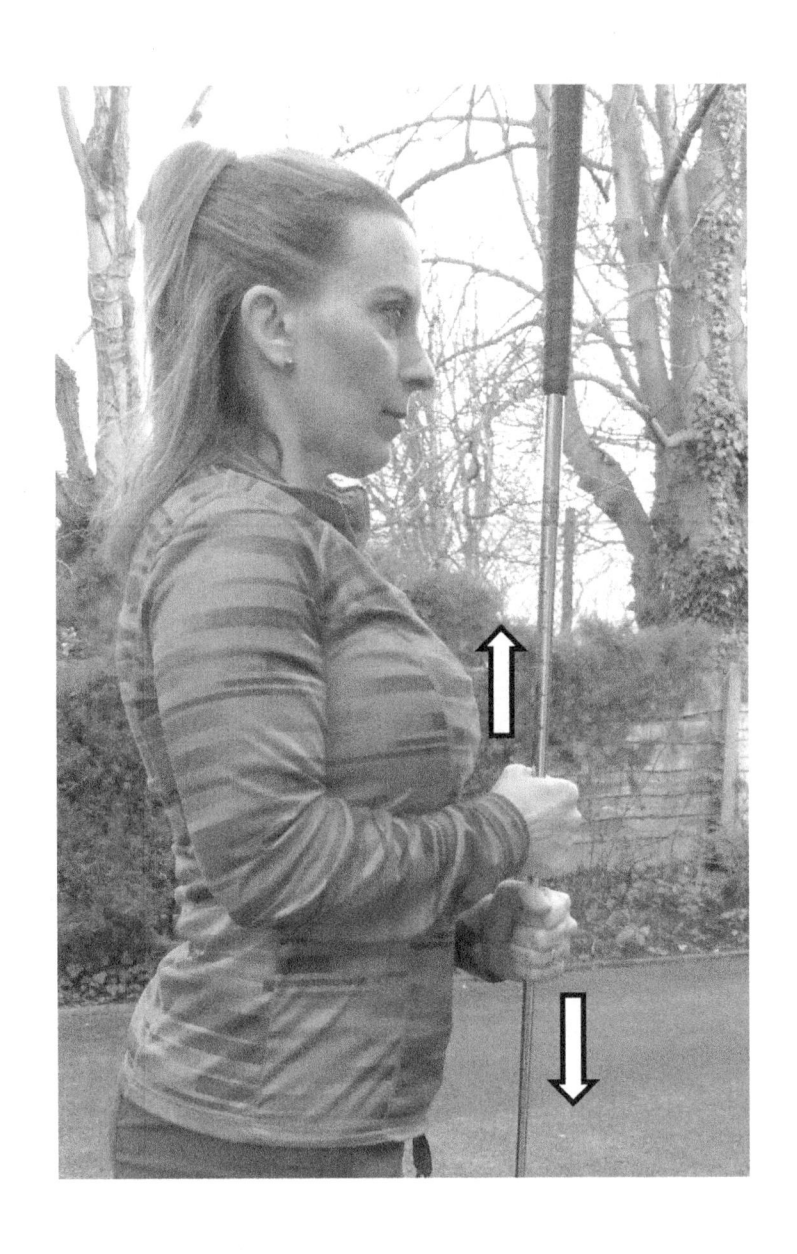

Arms – Upper Arm Triceps Overhead Press

Stand upright with the club held vertically behind your back. The supporting hand holds the club low behind the small of your back while the other arm being exercised holds the club overhead. The upper arm should be bent at approximately 90 degrees. In this position, the arms engage to pull the club in opposite directions, with the overhead hand/arm engaging the triceps muscles to do so.

The harder you engage the muscles, the more intense the exercise becomes, so be sure to exercise at a level of force and intensity that best suits your ability.

When you perform an isometric exercise, never hold your breath. Always breathe deeply and naturally, which will be about 10 full breaths in and out at a rate of about 1 second per full breath. Perform each exercise for no less than 7 seconds and no longer than 10. Be sure to exercise both arms evenly by reversing the procedure.

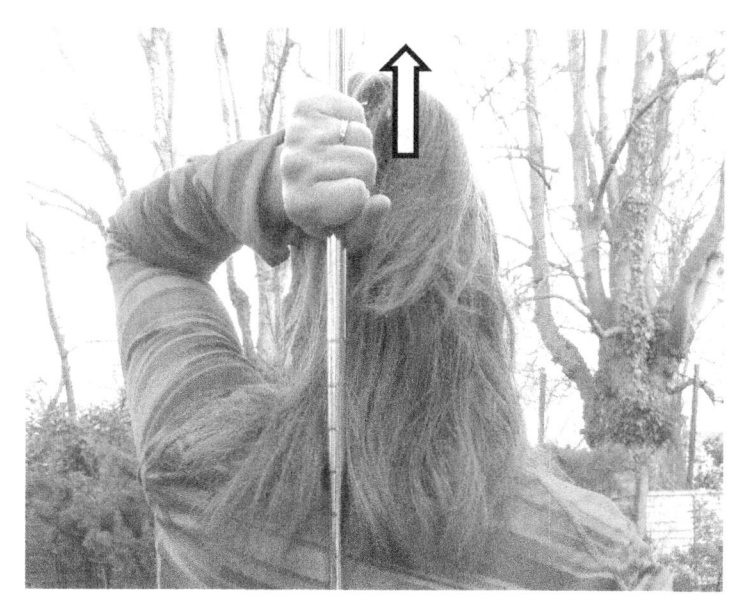

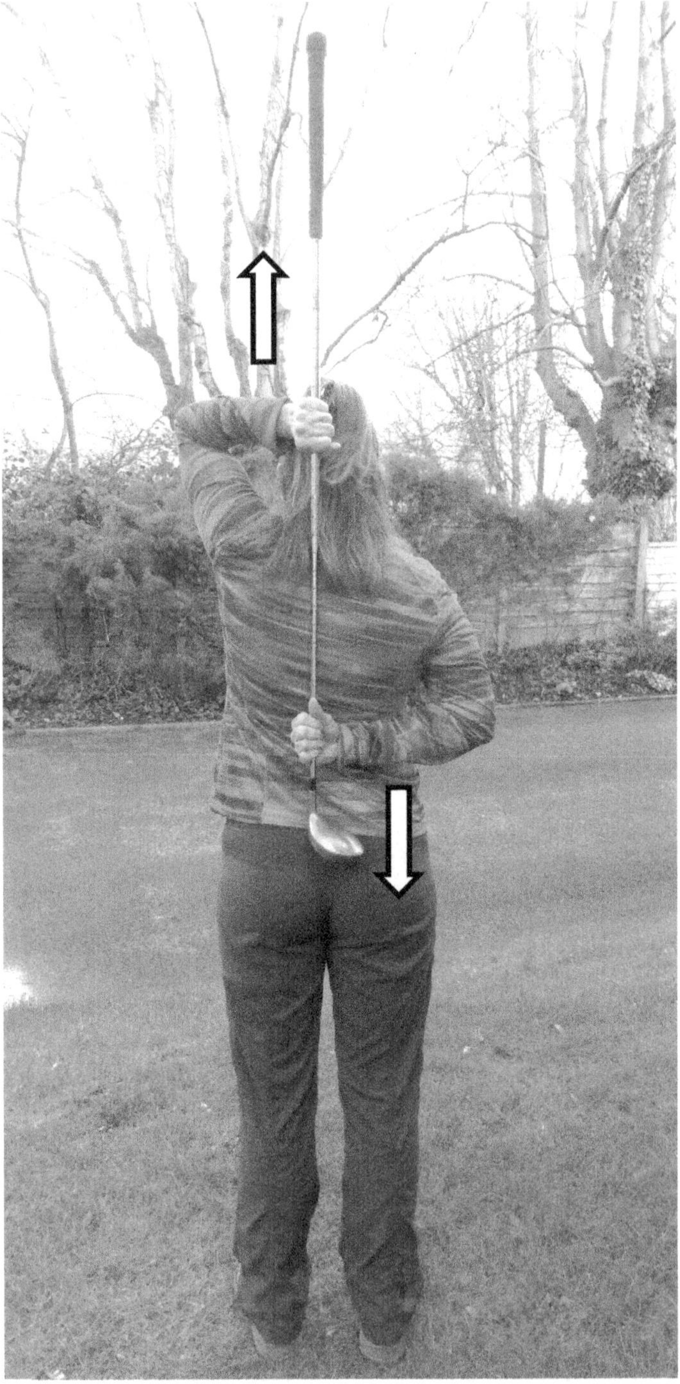

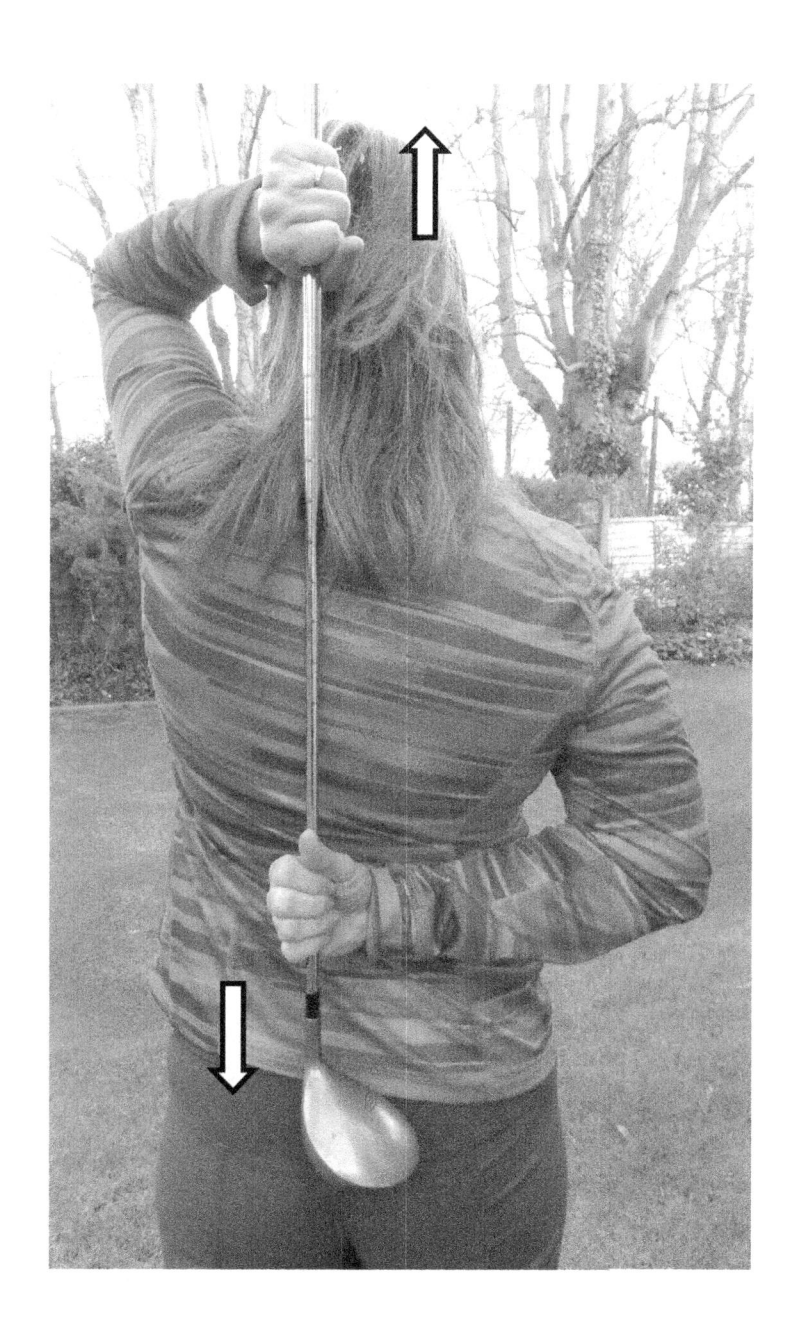

103

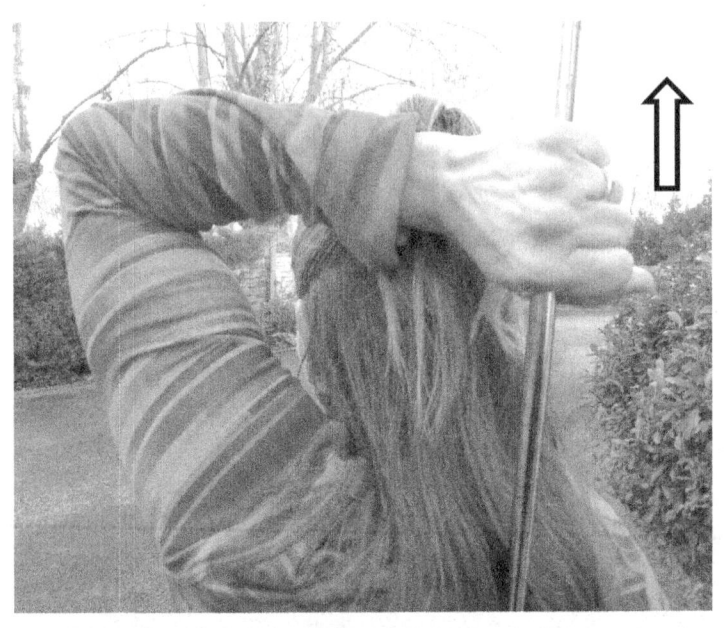

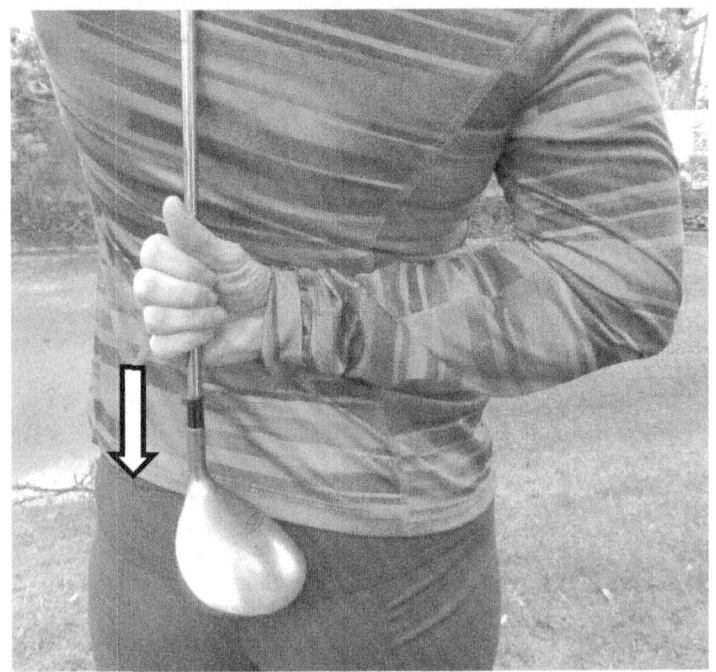

Arms – Upper Arm Triceps Press Down

Stand upright with the club held in one hand vertically in front of you on a firm surface. The arm should be bent at approximately 90 degrees, and you should grip either the handle sideways or over the top. Keep your elbow close to the body and press down to engage the rear upper arm triceps muscles as if you are trying to drive the club into the floor/ground.

The harder you engage the muscles, the more intense the exercise becomes, so be sure to exercise at a level of force and intensity that best suits your ability.

When you perform an isometric exercise, never hold your breath. Always breathe deeply and naturally, which will be about 10 full breaths in and out at a rate of about 1 second per full breath. Perform each exercise for no less than 7 seconds and no longer than 10. Be sure to exercise both arms evenly by reversing the procedure.

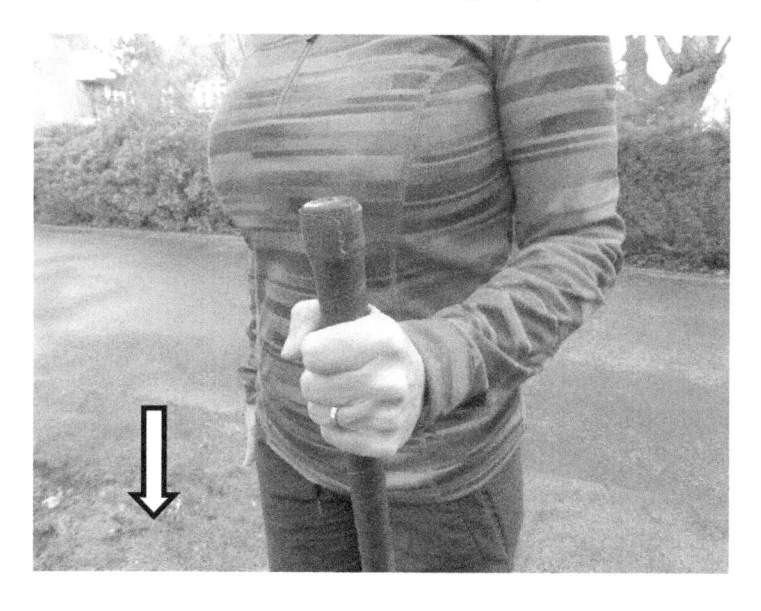

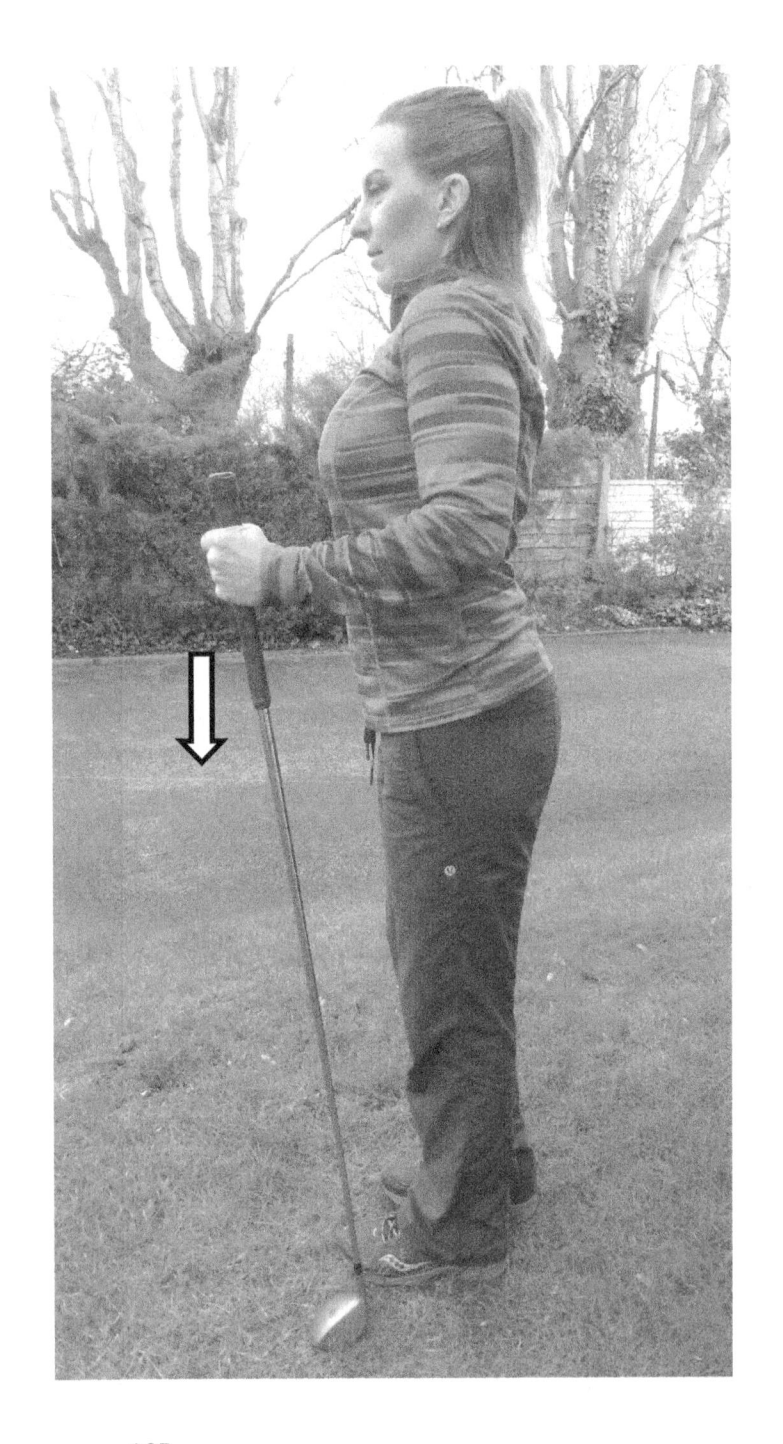

106

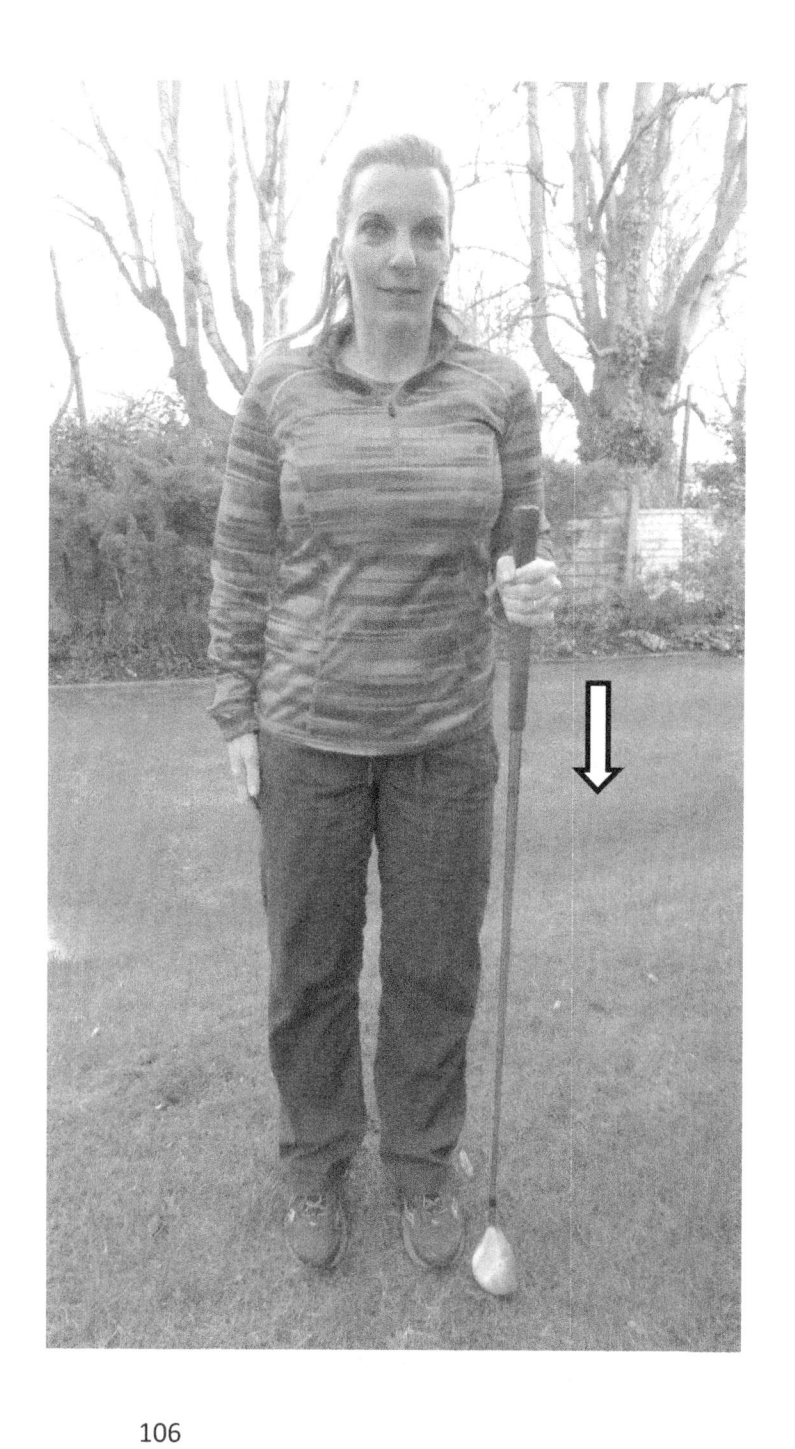

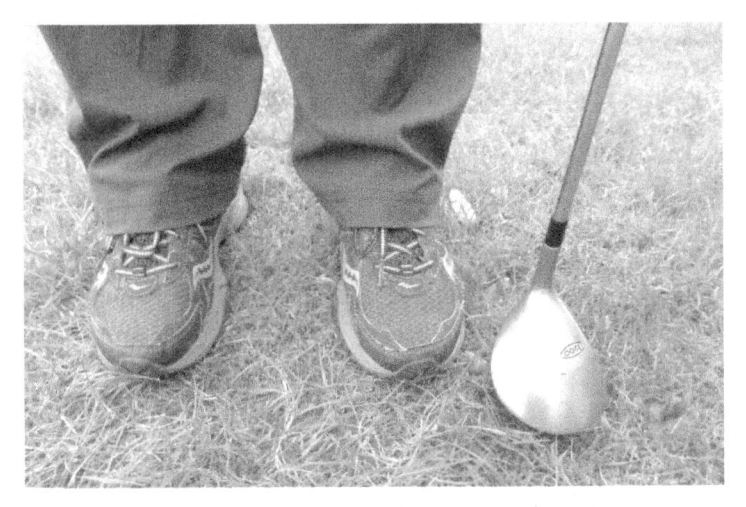

Always be sure to place the club on a solid surface.

To exercise both triceps/arms at the same time, simply place both hands over the handle of the club and perform the same exercise for both arms simultaneously.

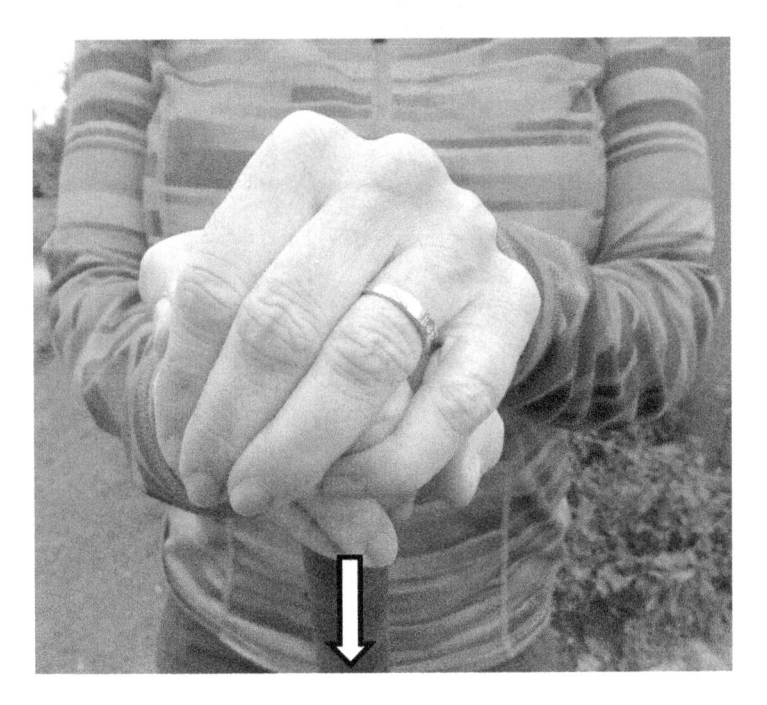

Arms – Forearms: Water Bottle Gripper

Ideally, you will need three pairs of plastic water bottles, each with a screw cap, making six bottles in total. Make certain that each pair of bottles is identical in size. The smallest size bottle should allow you to almost get your fingers wrapped completely around it, the middle size bottle should be big enough to get your fingers partially around, and the largest size should make it challenging to get your fingers wrapped around it. Fill the bottles to the brim with plain tap water and ensure, if possible, that there is no air gap. Since water cannot be compressed, it will perfectly counterbalance even the strongest grip that is applied. Start with the smallest bottle size and work your way up with each set of exercises. Stand upright and hold one bottle in each hand, with your hands and arms slightly away from the body. In this position, apply as much force with your grip as you try to compress and crush the bottle. The harder you engage the muscles, the more intense the exercise becomes, so always be sure to exercise at a level of force that best suits your current ability. When you perform an isometric exercise, never hold your breath. Always breathe deeply and naturally, which will be about 10 full breaths in and out at a rate of about 1 second per full breath. Perform each exercise for no less than 7 seconds and no longer than 10. **NOTE: Do not use a glass bottle, a can, or a plastic bottle filled with carbonated liquid, as any of these may burst or shatter. We chose to only use one large bottle because of its weight when filled with liquid. The bottle can be used to exercise each hand individually, or if it is big enough and/or your hands are small enough, then both hands at the same time.**

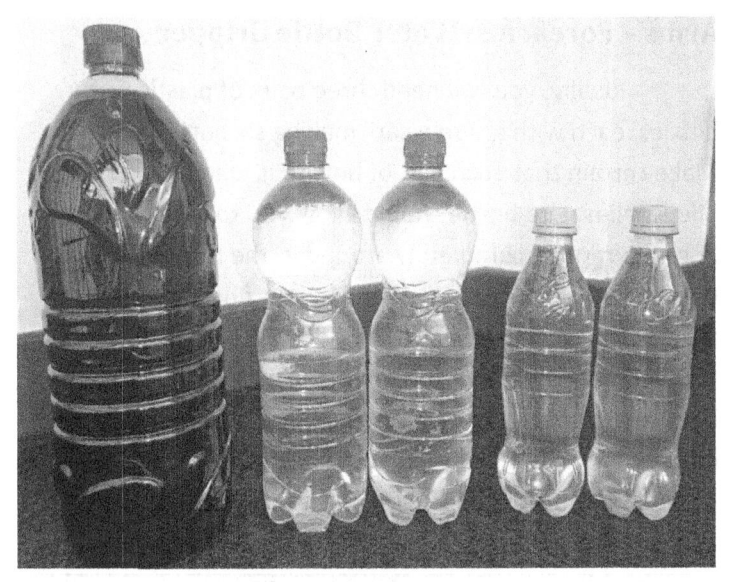

TOP: Forearm grip exercise bottles, large, medium, and small – Left to Right.

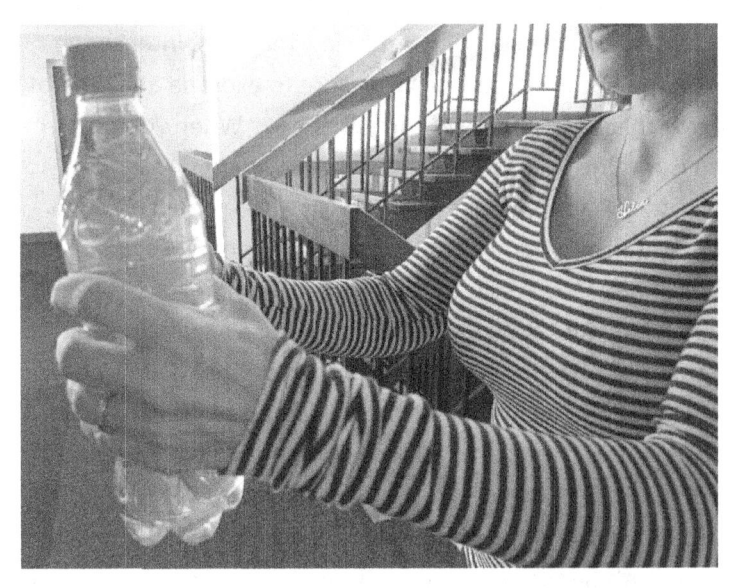

BOTTOM: Forearm grip exercise 1) Small bottles

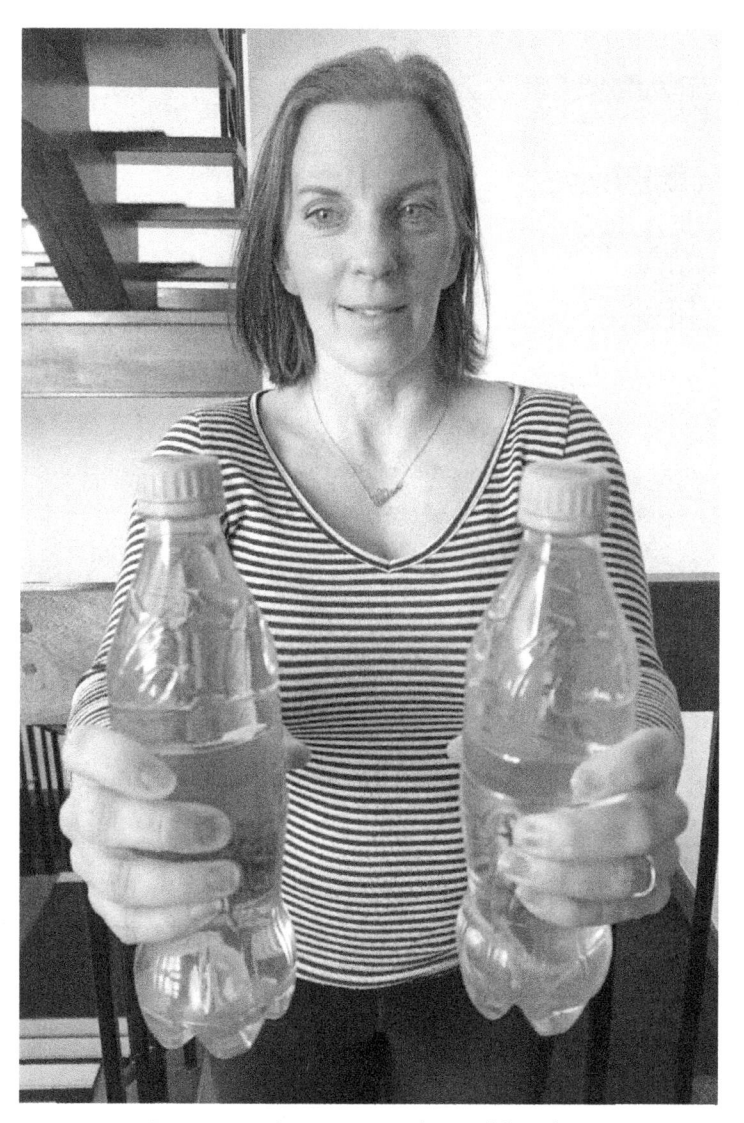

Forearm grip exercise 1) Small bottles

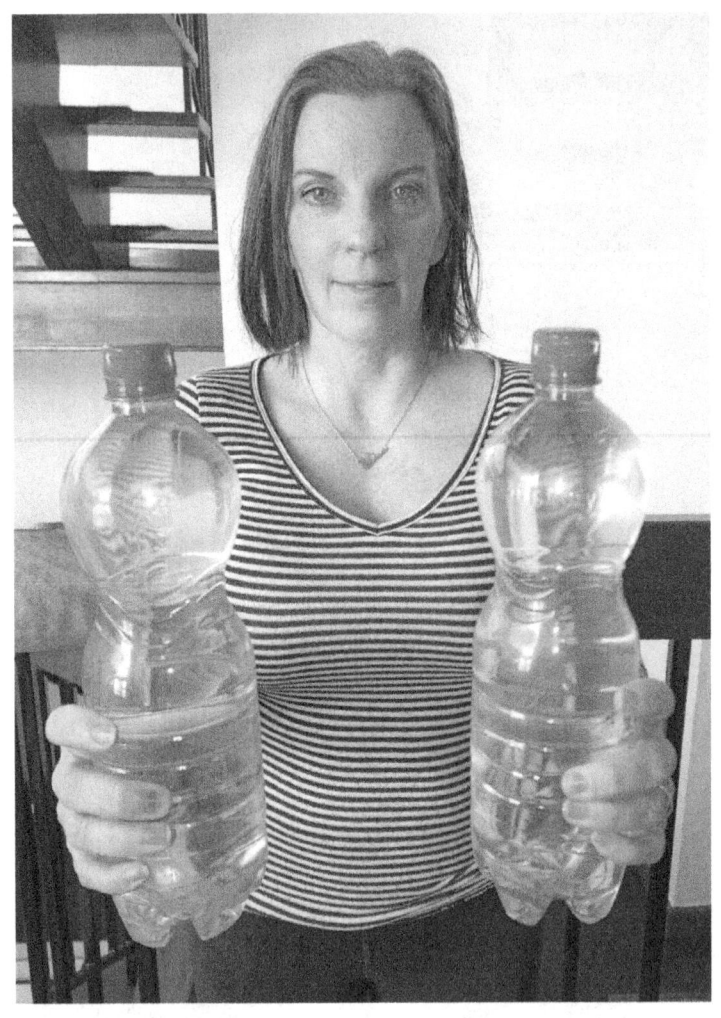

Forearm grip exercise 2) Medium bottles

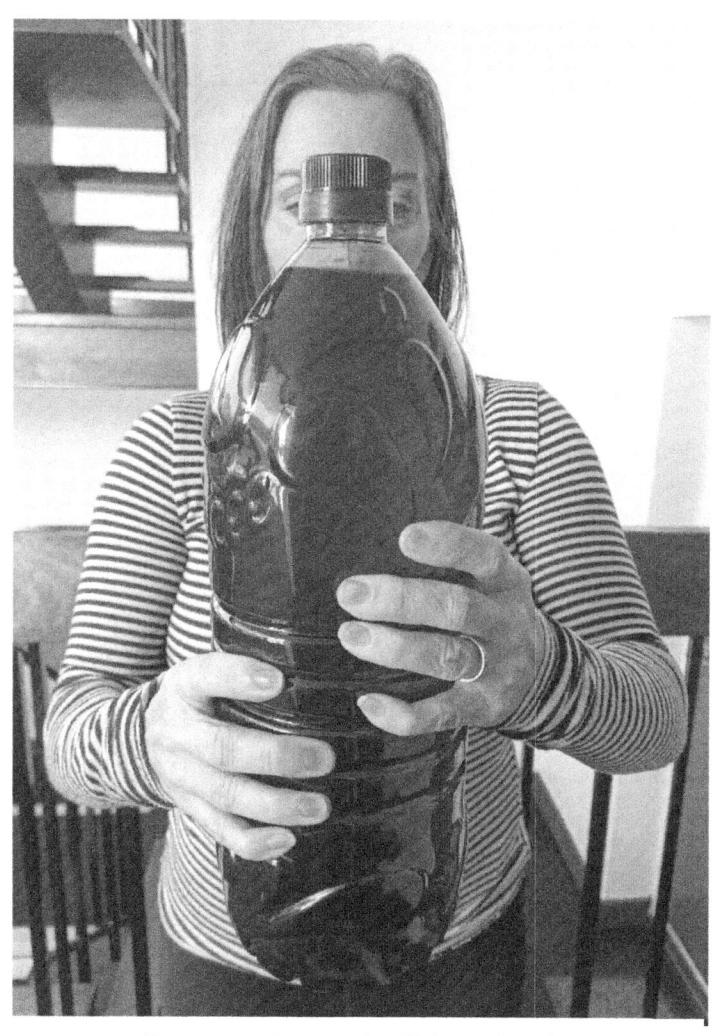

Forearm grip exercise 3) Large bottle
Both hands.

Lower Back – Good Morning Bend - Arms Back

Stand with your feet approximately shoulder-width apart and with your knees slightly bent. Bend forward only from the hip, keep the back straight and hold the club behind you with both arms extended as far as possible. If you are able to do so, keep the club raised so that it does not rest on your backside/hips. In that position, be sure to engage the lower back and buttock muscles to perform the exercise.

The harder you engage the muscles, the more intense the exercise becomes, so always be sure to exercise at a level of force and intensity that best suits your ability.

When you perform an isometric exercise, never hold your breath. Always breathe deeply and naturally, which will be about 10 full breaths in and out at a rate of about 1 second per full breath. Perform each exercise for no less than 7 seconds and no longer than 10.

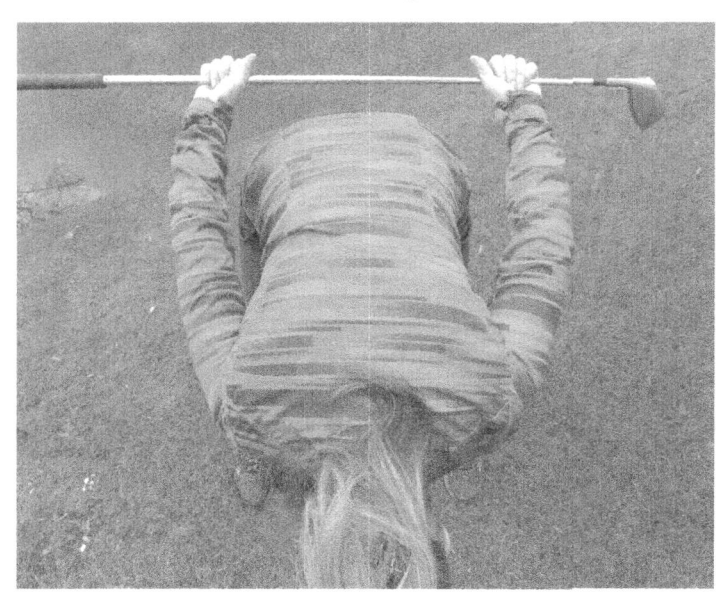

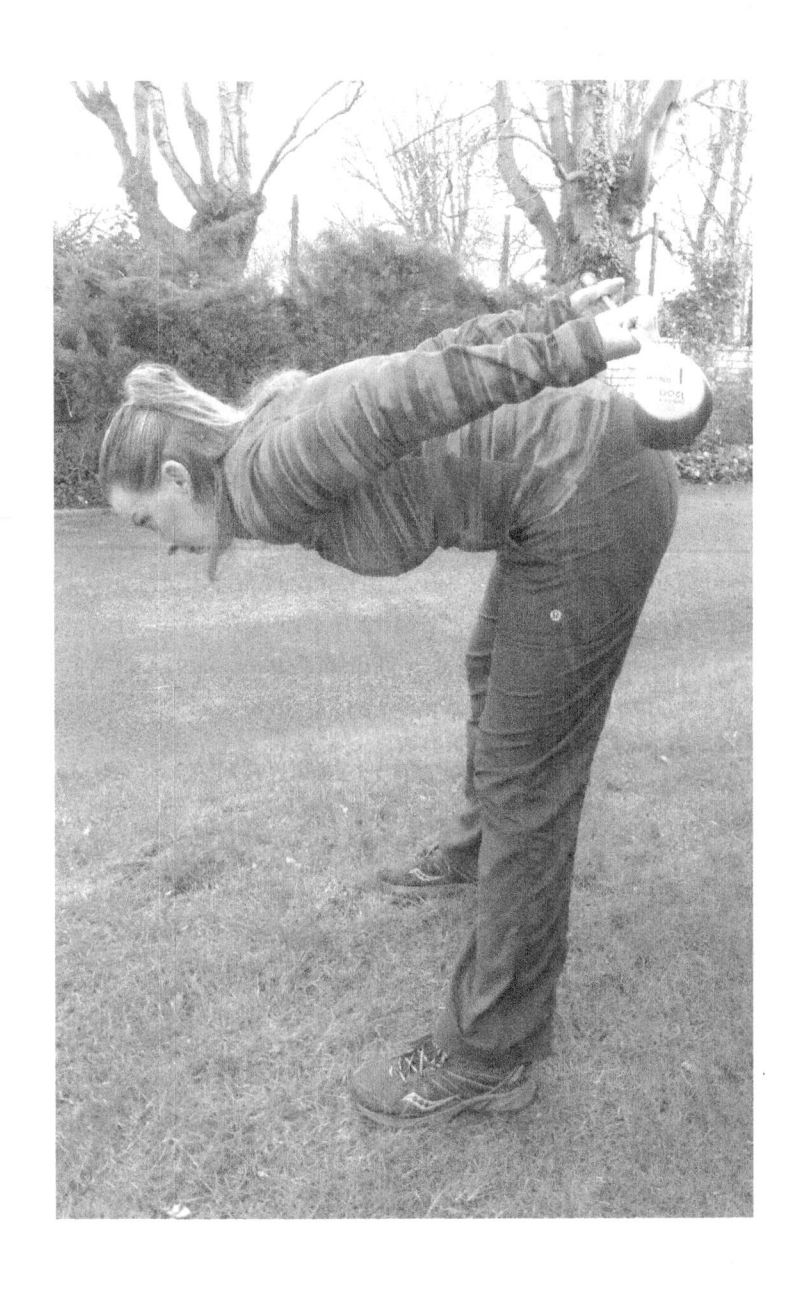

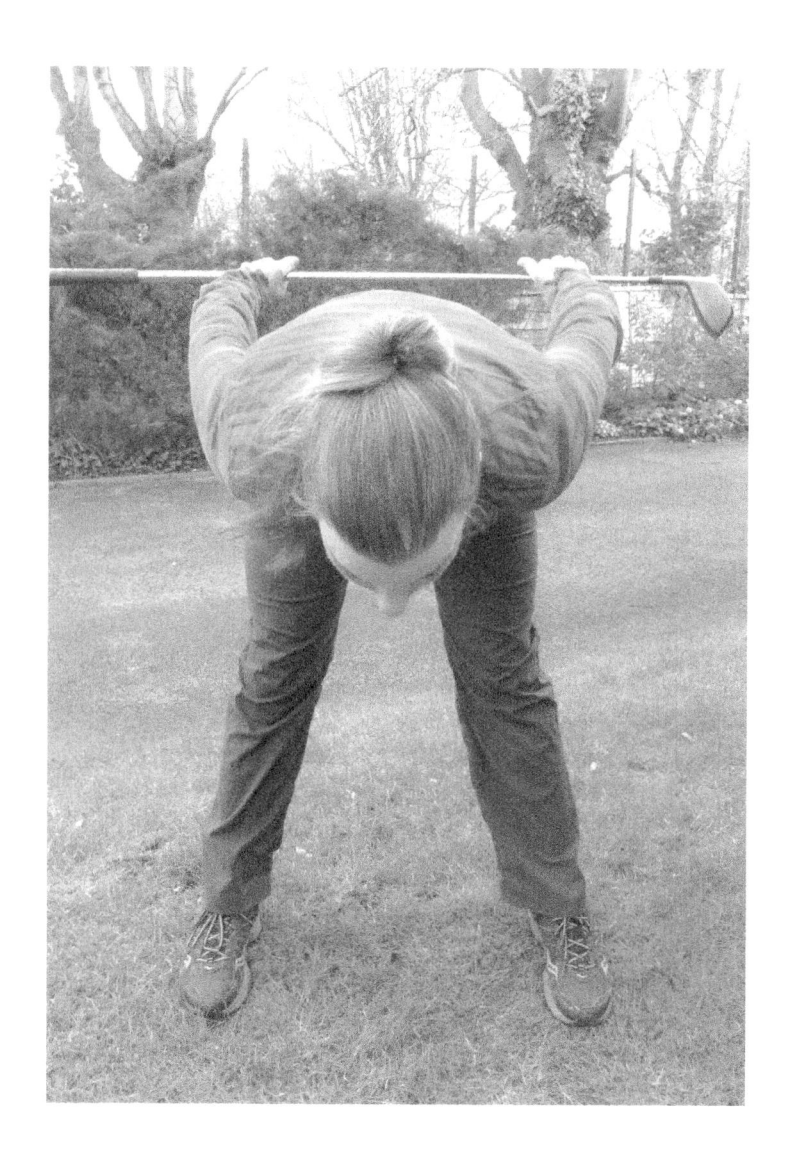

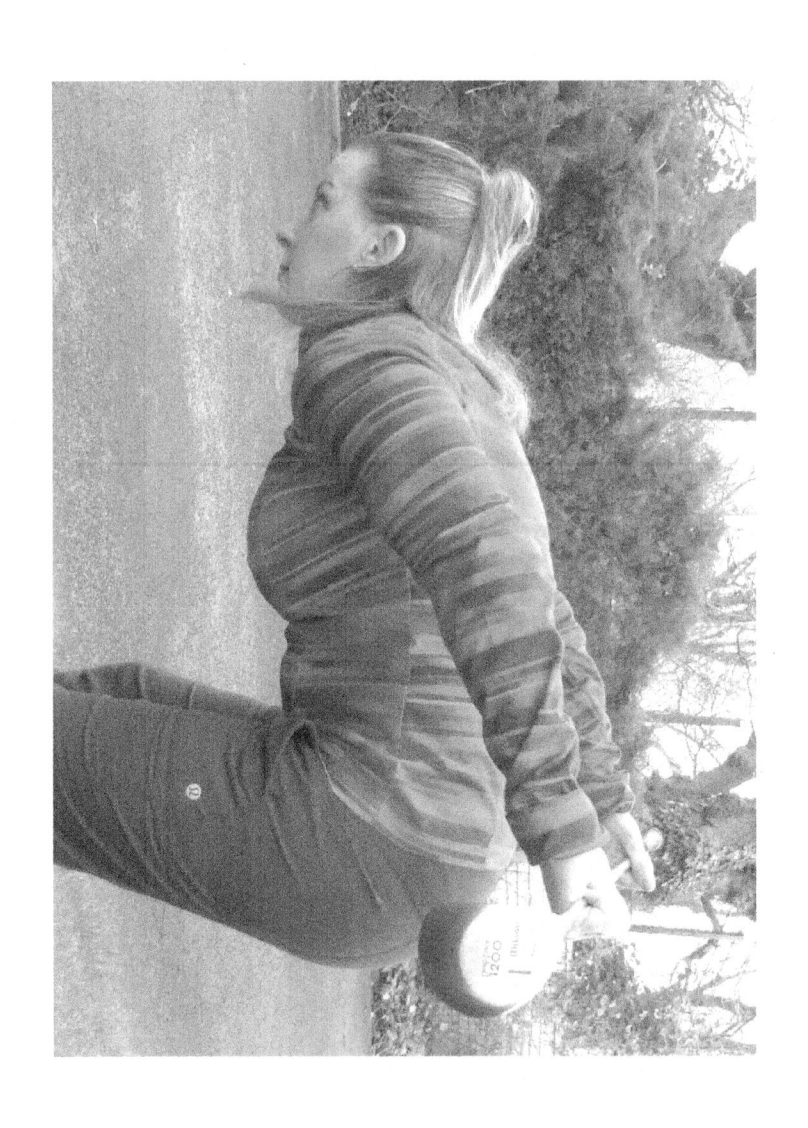

Lower Back – Good Morning - Arms Forward

NOTE: This exercise is more challenging than the previous exercise with the arms extended to the rear, as both arms must be extended forward.

Stand with your feet approximately shoulder-width apart and with your knees slightly bent. Bend forward only from the hip and keep the back straight, then extend both arms horizontally in front of you to align with the near-horizontal level of your back. Hold the club at about should-width apart as you engage the lower back and buttock muscles to perform the exercise. At the same time, apply pressure to pull the golf club apart. The harder you engage the muscles, the more intense the exercise becomes, so always be sure to exercise at a level of force and intensity that best suits your ability. When you perform an isometric exercise, never hold your breath. Always breathe deeply and naturally, which will be about 10 full breaths in and out at a rate of about 1 second per full breath. Perform each exercise for no less than 7 seconds and no longer than 10.

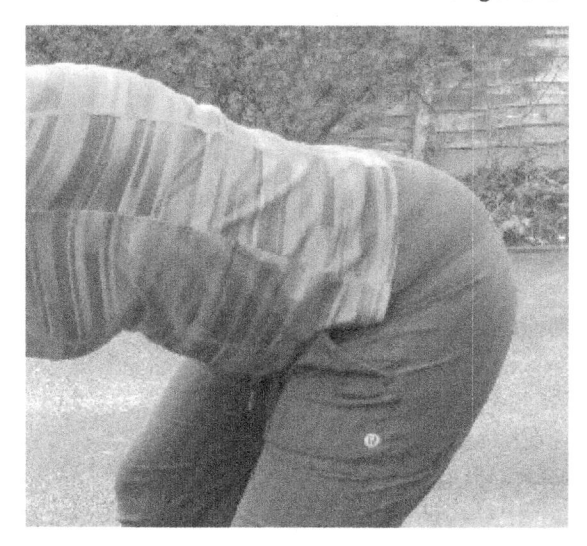

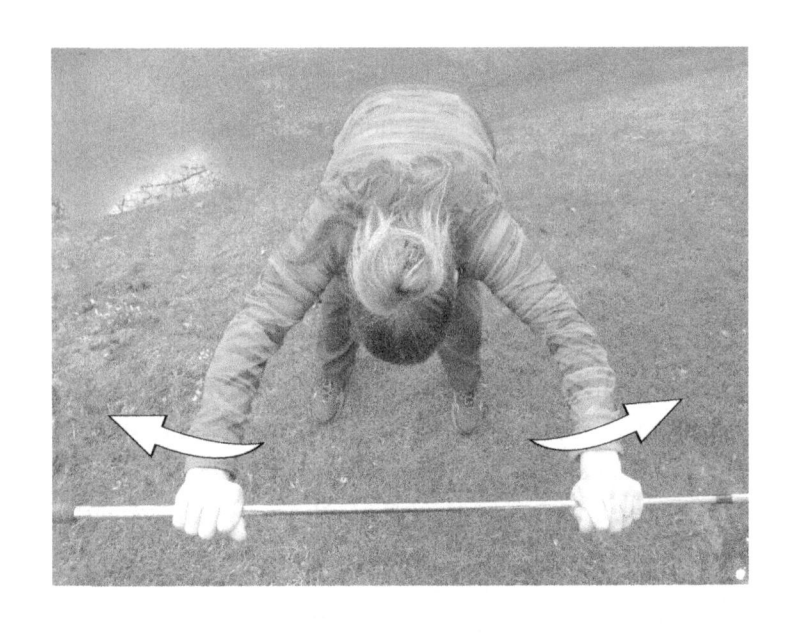

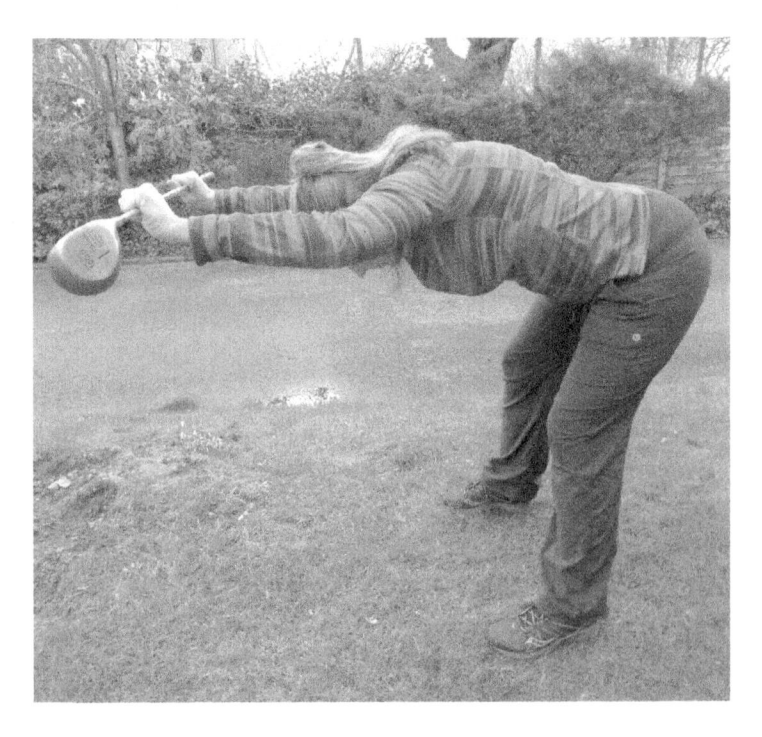

Upper Back – Chest Height Club Pull-Apart

Stand upright with your feet approximately shoulder-width apart. Hold the club in front of you at chest height and grip the club firmly. The hand position can vary according to your preference. It can range from close, where both hands touch, and wide, where the hands are wider than shoulder-width apart. Each position has merit and will exercise the muscles in a different position, so the choice is yours. Be sure to vary the hand position in each workout session you perform. In this position, apply pressure to pull the club apart. This will engage the muscles of the upper back. The harder you engage the muscles, the more intense the exercise becomes, so always be sure to exercise at a level of force and intensity that best suits your ability. When you perform an isometric exercise, never hold your breath. Always breathe deeply and naturally, which will be about 10 full breaths in and out at a rate of about 1 second per full breath. Perform each exercise for no less than 7 seconds and no longer than 10.

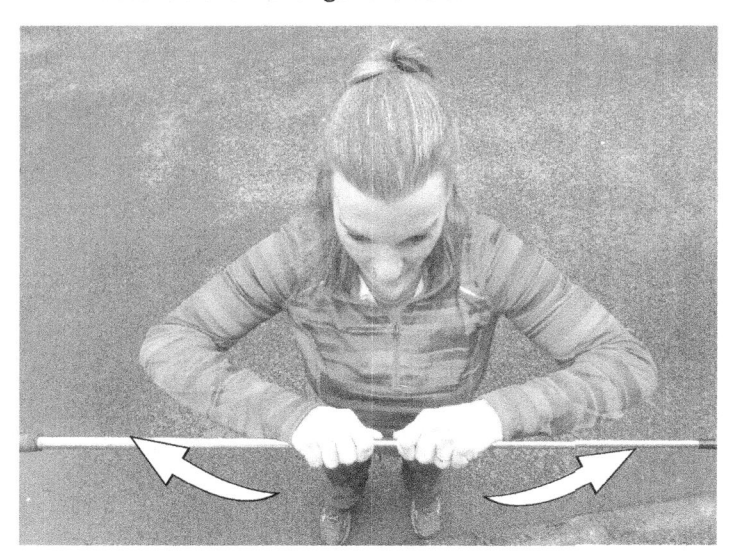

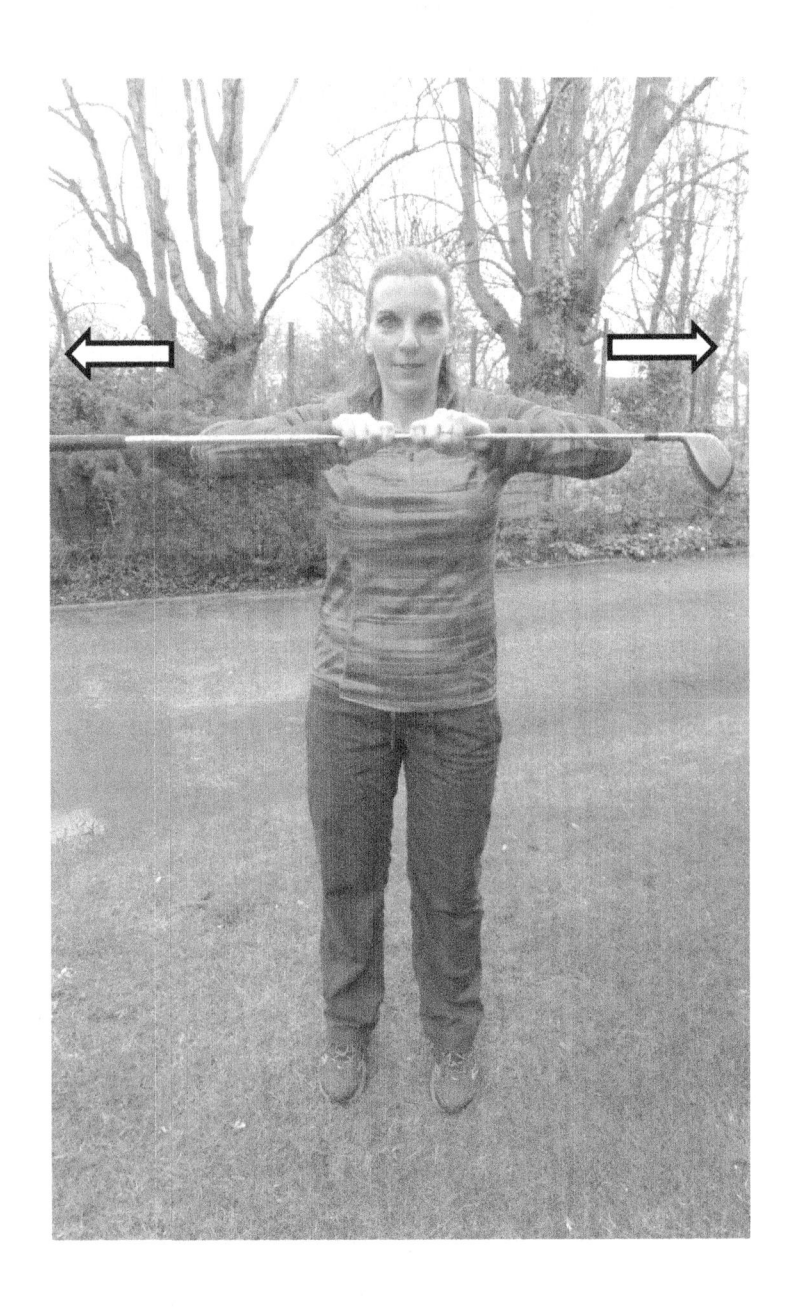

Upper Back – Overhead Club Pull-Apart

Stand with your feet approximately shoulder-width apart. Hold the club as near to horizontal as possible above your head with your hands gripping it approximately shoulder-width apart and with your arms slightly bent. Keep your arms locked in that slightly bent position throughout the exercise. In that position, engage the upper back muscles by trying to pull the club apart above your head.

The harder you engage the muscles, the more intense the exercise becomes, so always be sure to exercise at a level of force and intensity that best suits your ability.

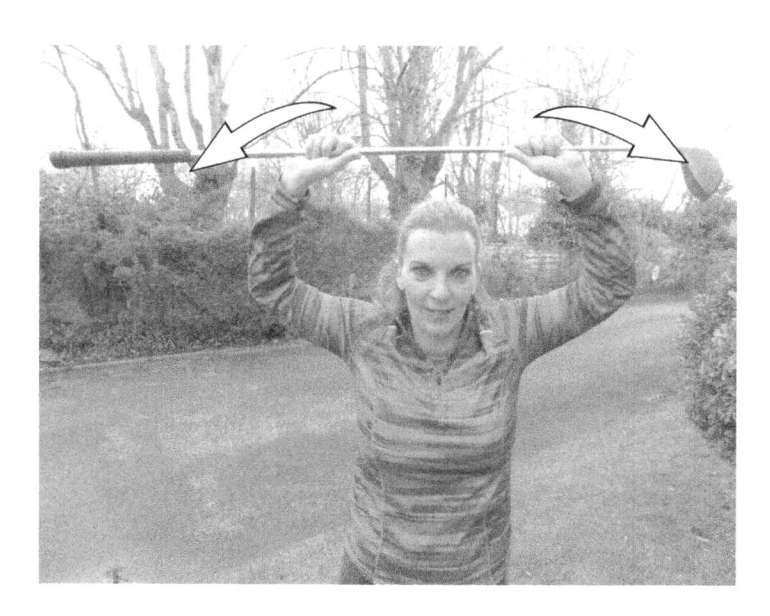

When you perform an isometric exercise, never hold your breath. Always breathe deeply and naturally, which will be about 10 full breaths in and out at a rate of about 1 second per full breath. Perform each exercise for no less than 7 seconds and no longer than 10.

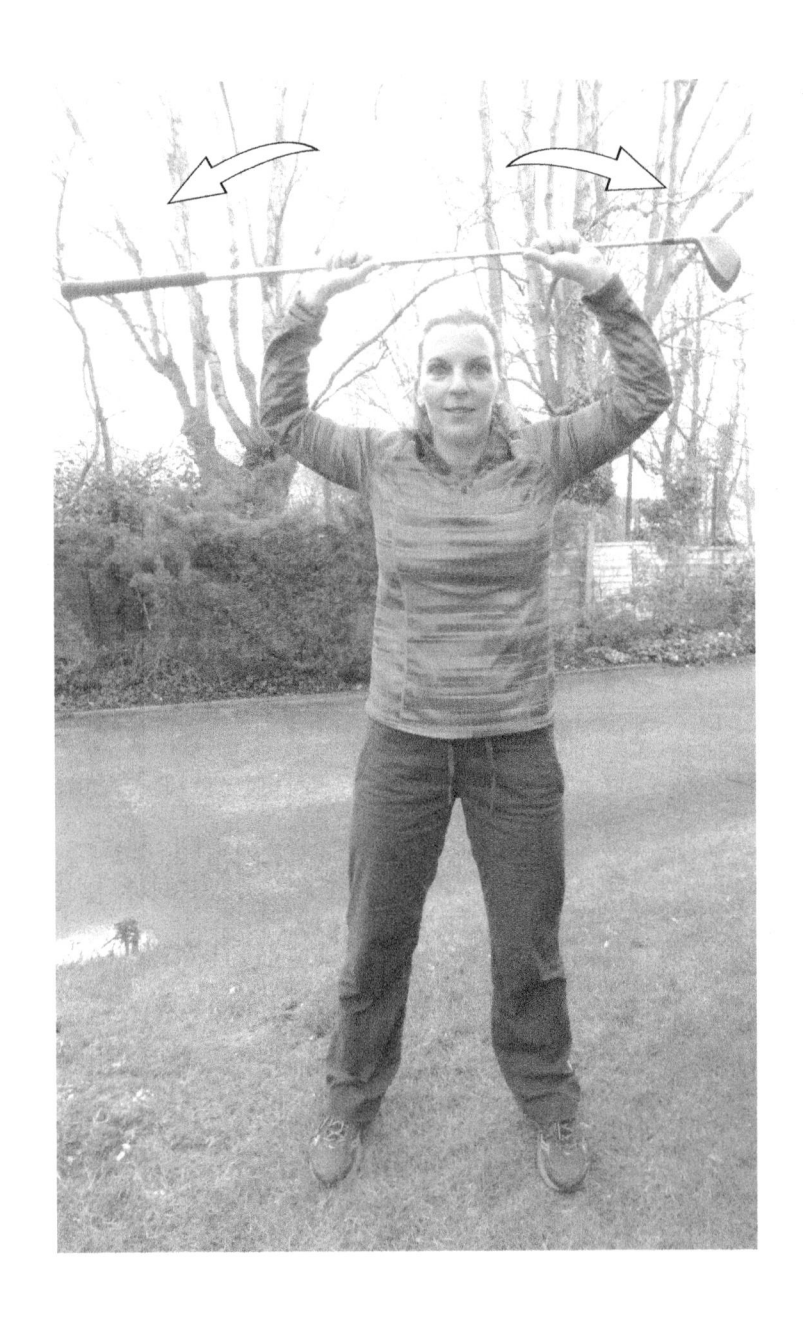

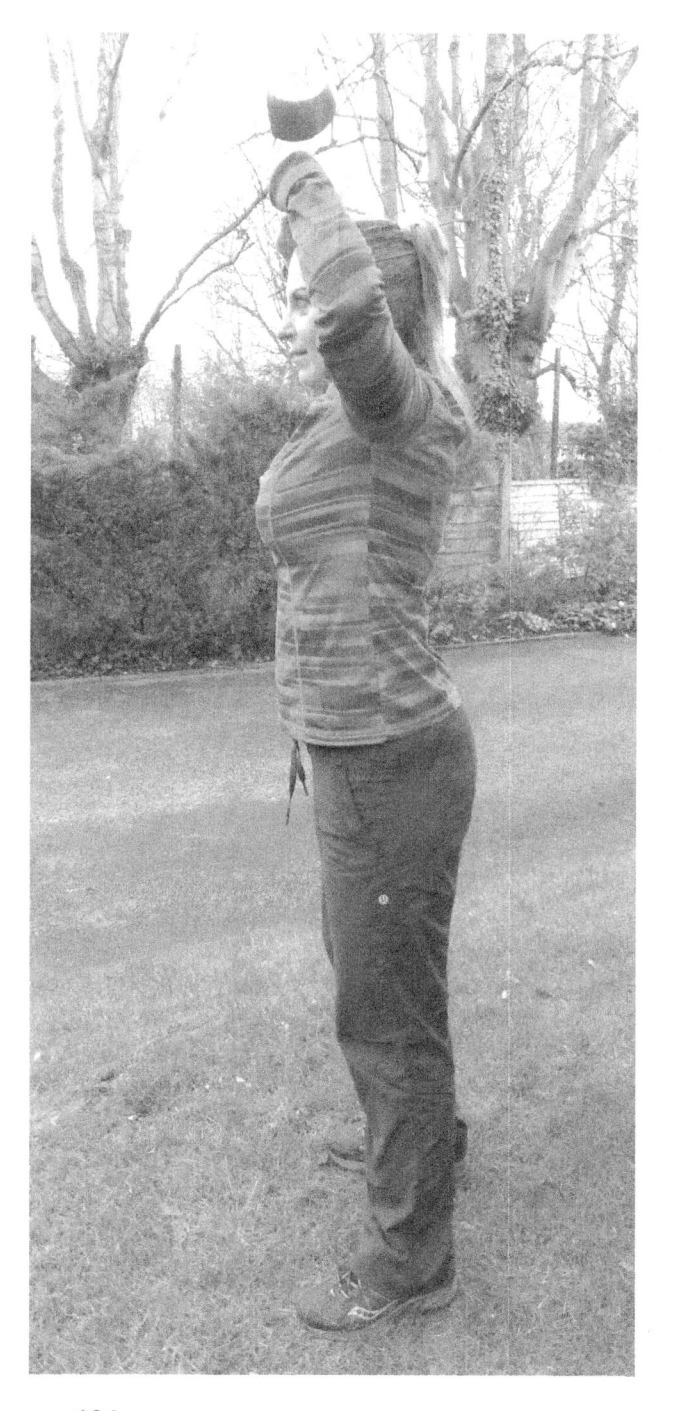

NOTE: Adjust the hand position along the length of the club as needed. Positioning the hands either closer together or further apart will exercise the upper back muscles at different points.

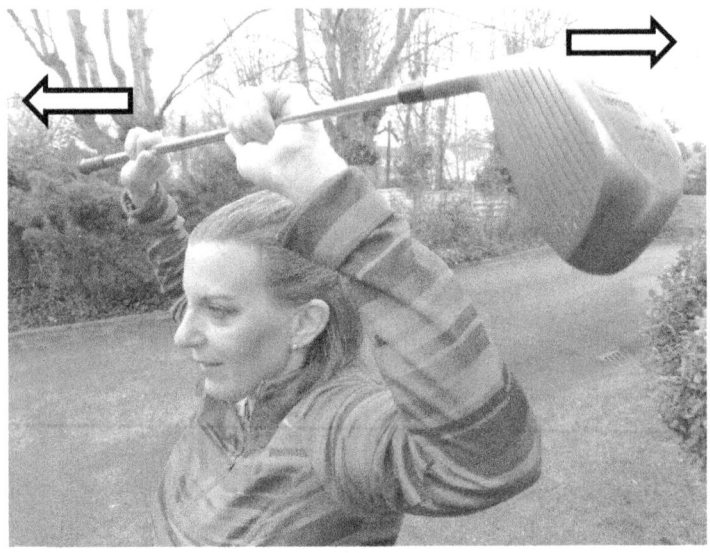

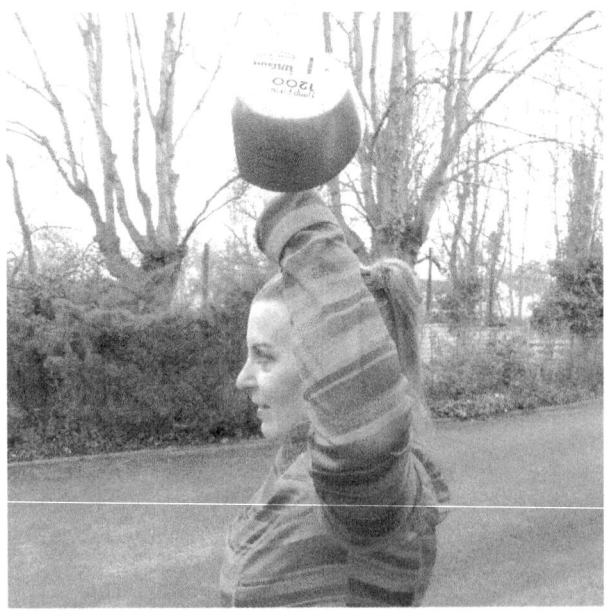

Upper Back – Behind Back Club-Push Together

Stand upright with your feet approximately shoulder-width apart. Hold the club behind your back at waist height and grip with your hands approximately shoulder-width apart. Keep your arms slightly bent and locked in this position throughout the exercise, and be sure to hold the club slightly away from your body. Apply pressure to push the club inward as if trying to compress it so that your hands will eventually meet. This will engage the muscles of the upper back.

The harder you engage the muscles, the more intense the exercise becomes, so always be sure to exercise at a level of force and intensity that best suits your ability.

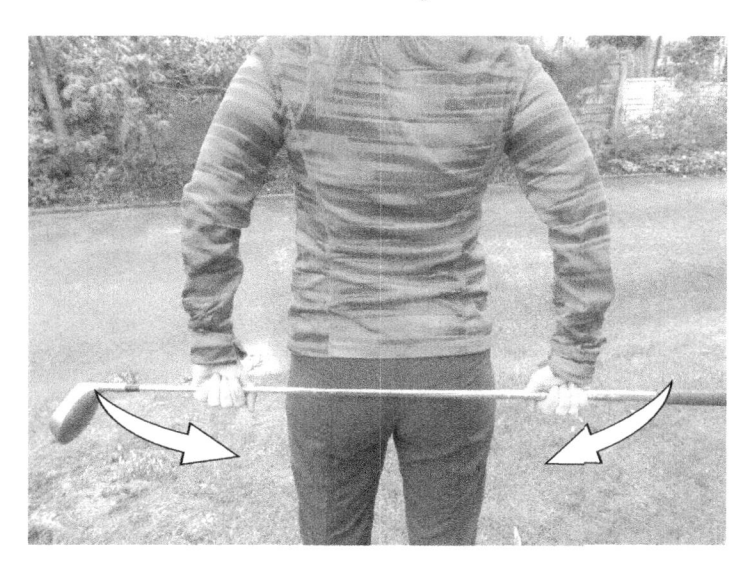

When you perform an isometric exercise, never hold your breath. Always breathe deeply and naturally, which will be about 10 full breaths in and out at a rate of about 1 second per full breath. Perform each exercise for no less than 7 seconds and no longer than 10.

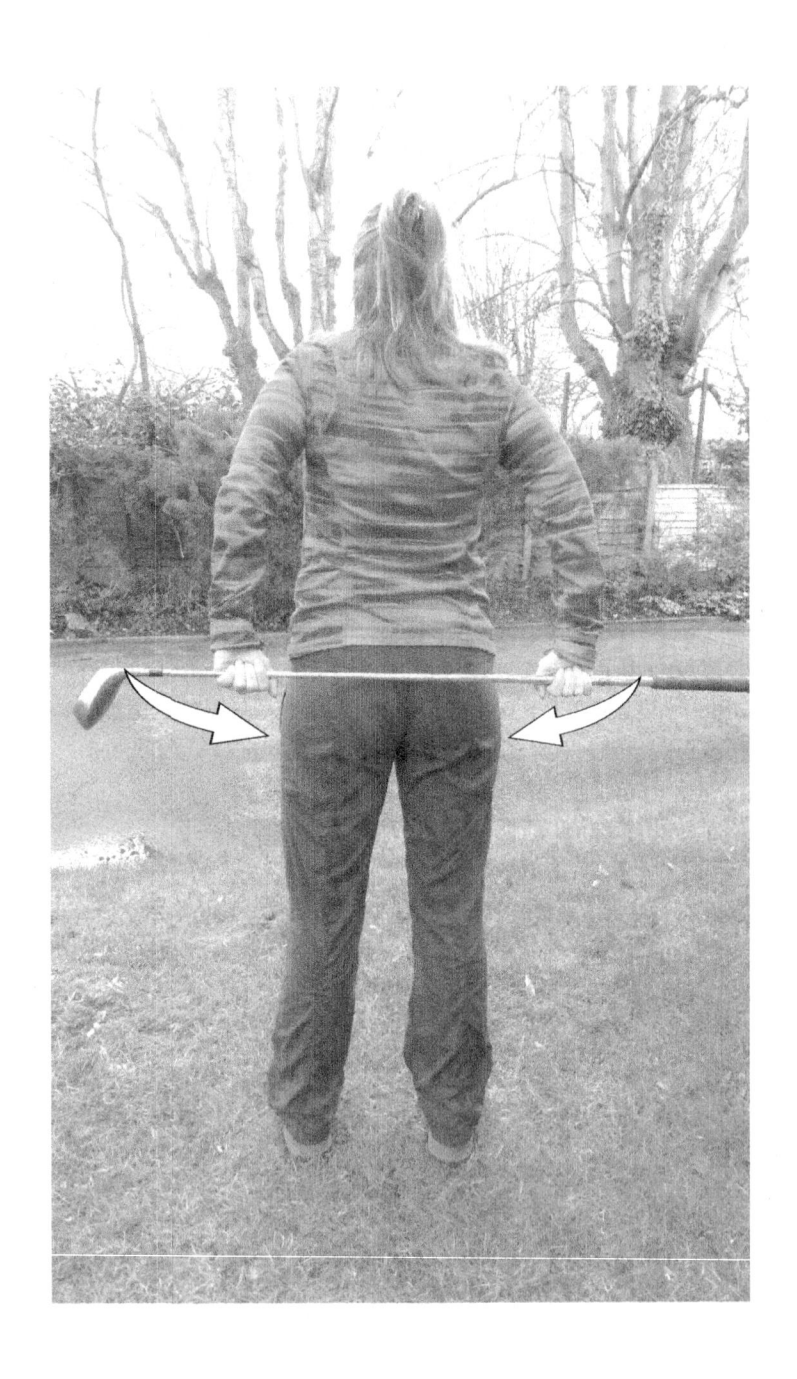

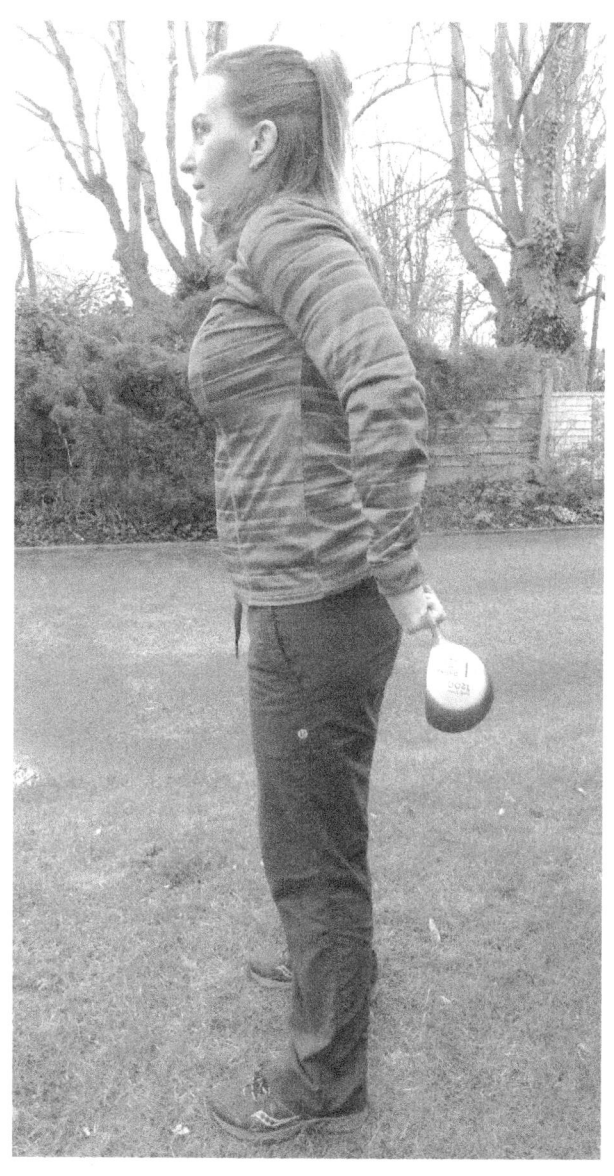

NOTE: Adjust the hand position along the length of the club as needed. Positioning the hands either closer together or further apart will exercise the upper back muscles at different points.

Upper Back – Single Arm Row Club on Floor

Position one foot and leg slightly forward in a short lunge stance. Bend forward slightly from the hips, keeping the back straight as you do. Make sure that the club is on solid ground and will not slip. Hold the upper end of the club or the handle in front of you with your arms slightly bent and locked in that position. Apply pressure in this position as you attempt to perform a single-arm rowing action to drive the club down and backward, even though the club will not move. This will engage the muscles of the upper back. Be sure to exercise both sides of the body.

The harder you engage the muscles, the more intense the exercise becomes, so always be sure to exercise at a level of force and intensity that best suits your ability. When you perform an isometric exercise, never hold your breath. Always breathe deeply and naturally, which will be about 10 full breaths in and out at a rate of about 1 second per full breath. Perform each exercise for no less than 7 seconds and no longer than 10.

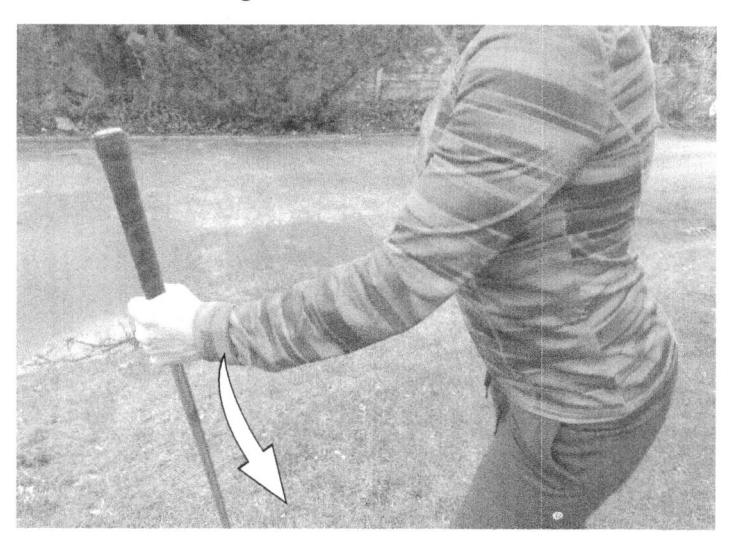

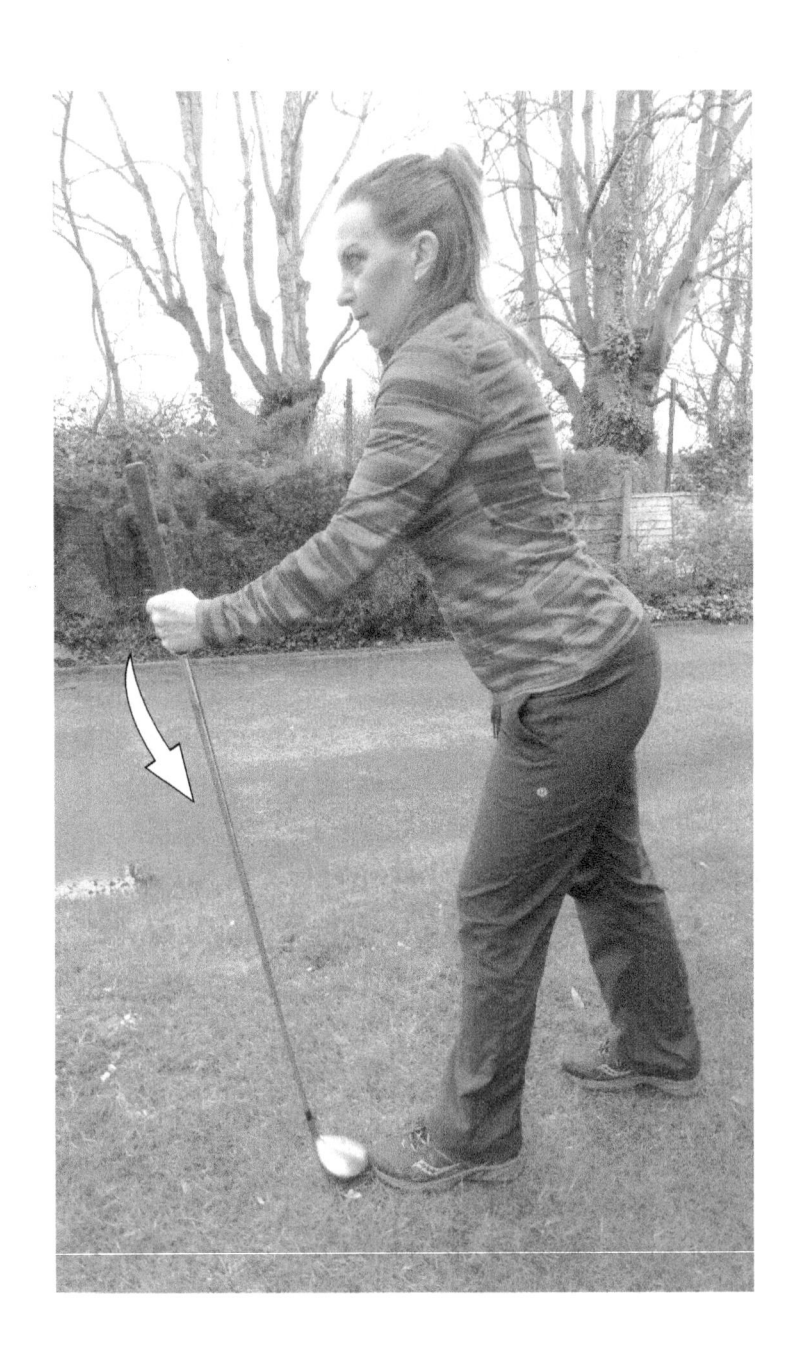

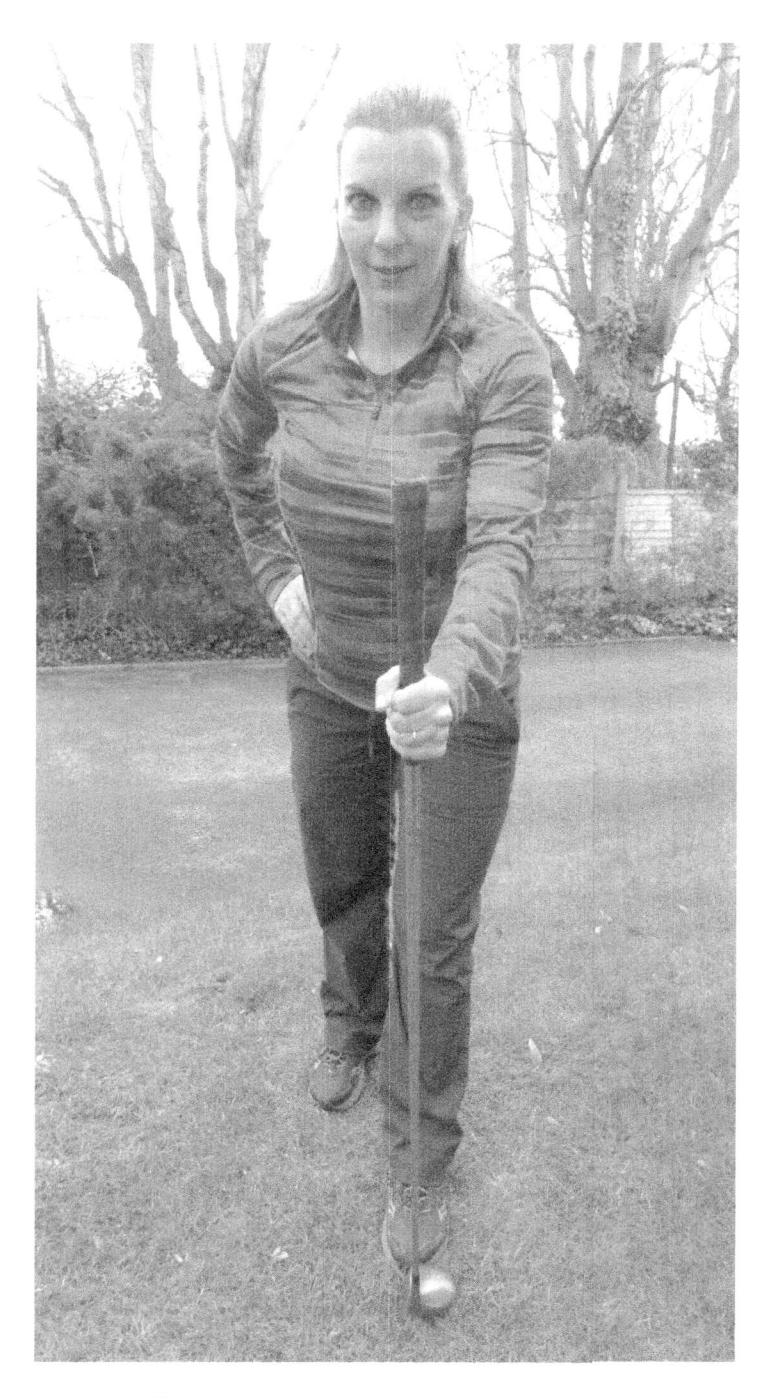

TIP: If the ground is soft or if you are unsure about the possibility of the club slipping during the exercise, lock the tip of the club on the ground in front of your shoe. This way, your shoe will act as an anchor point.

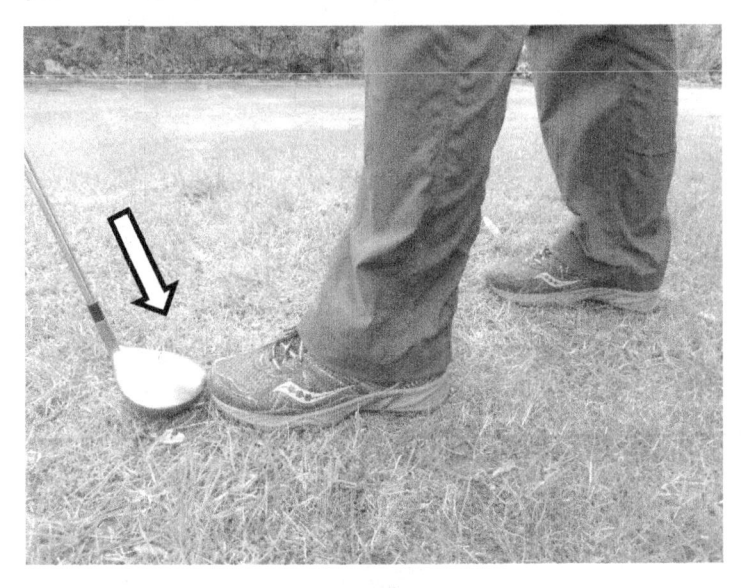

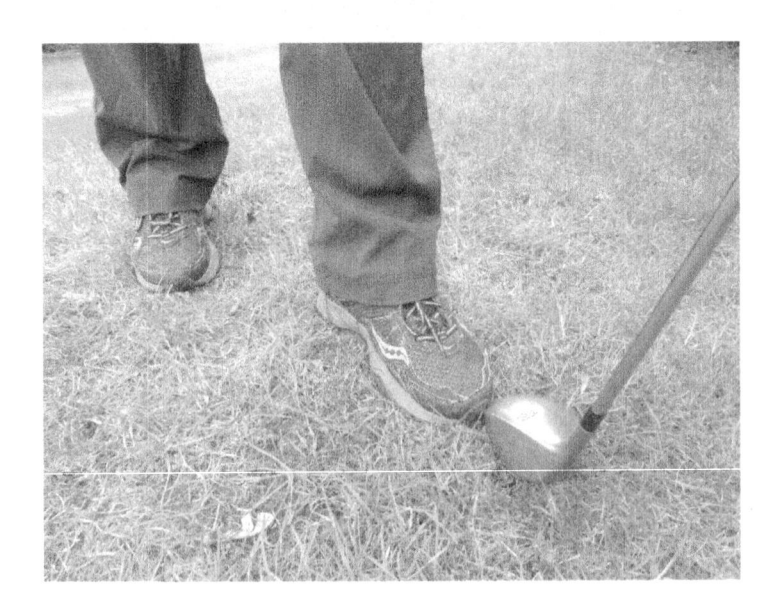

Upper Back – Single Arm Row Club Held Across Hip

Position one foot and leg slightly forward in a short lunge stance. Bend forward slightly from the hips, keeping the back straight as you do. Hold the upper end of the club or the handle in front of you with your arms slightly bent and locked in that position. Hold the lower end of the club in your other hand with your arm placed across your body/hips. This should secure the club roughly at hip height and at a slightly more acute angle than in the previous rowing exercise. This will engage the muscles of the upper back. Be sure to exercise both sides of the body.

The harder you engage the muscles, the more intense the exercise becomes, so always be sure to exercise at a level of force and intensity that best suits your ability. When you perform an isometric exercise, never hold your breath. Always breathe deeply and naturally, which will be about 10 full breaths in and out at a rate of about 1 second per full breath. Perform each exercise for no less than 7 seconds and no longer than 10.

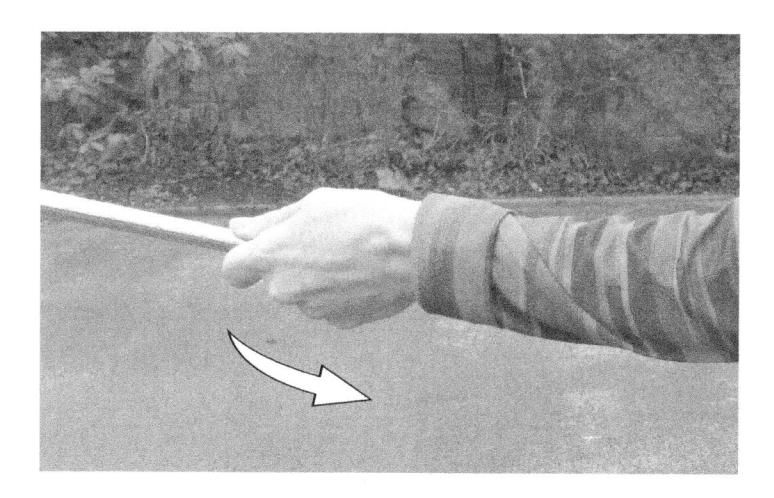

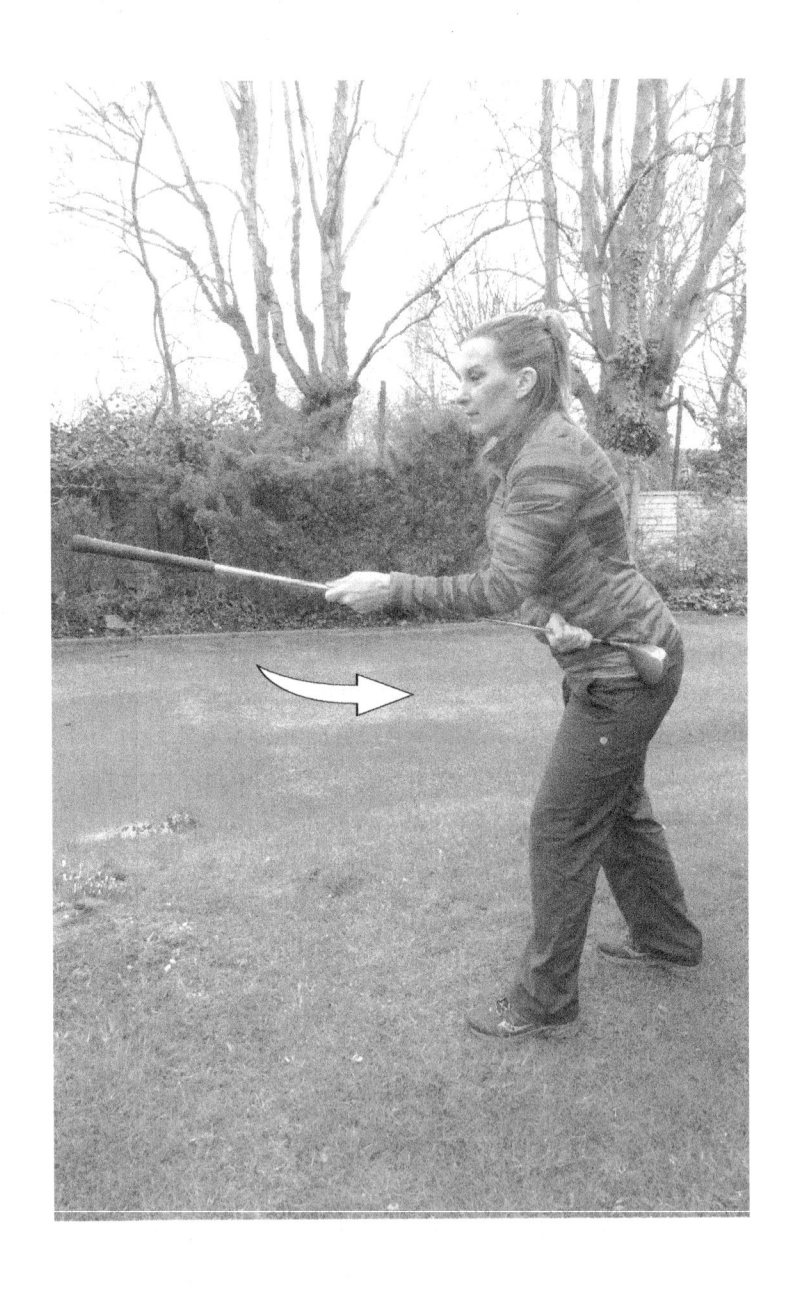

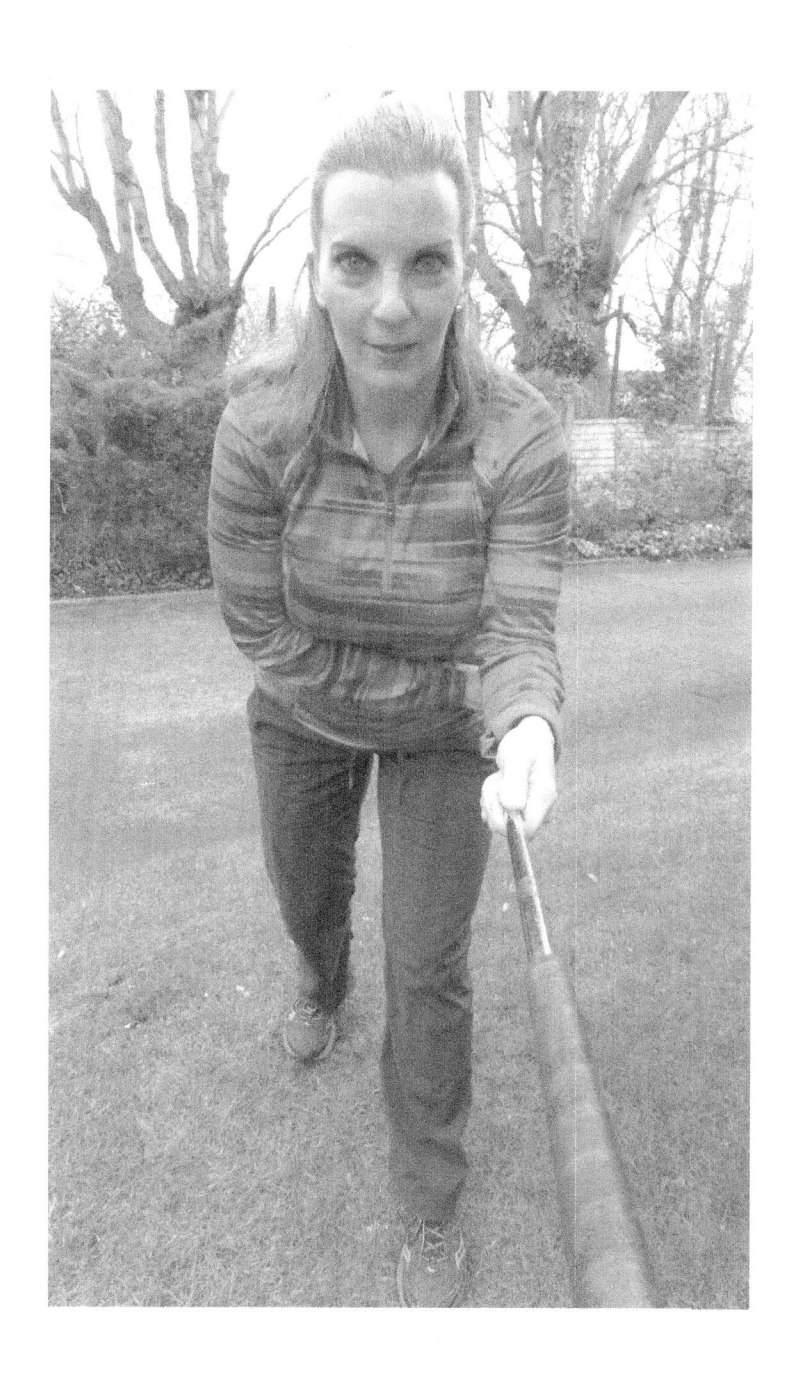

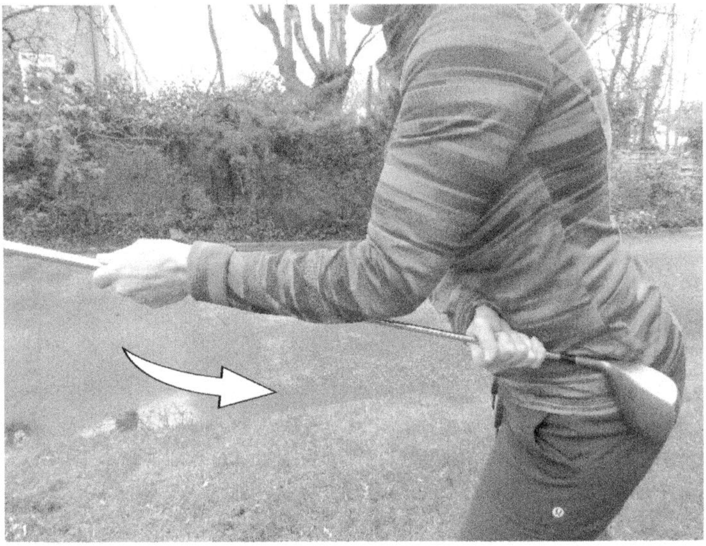

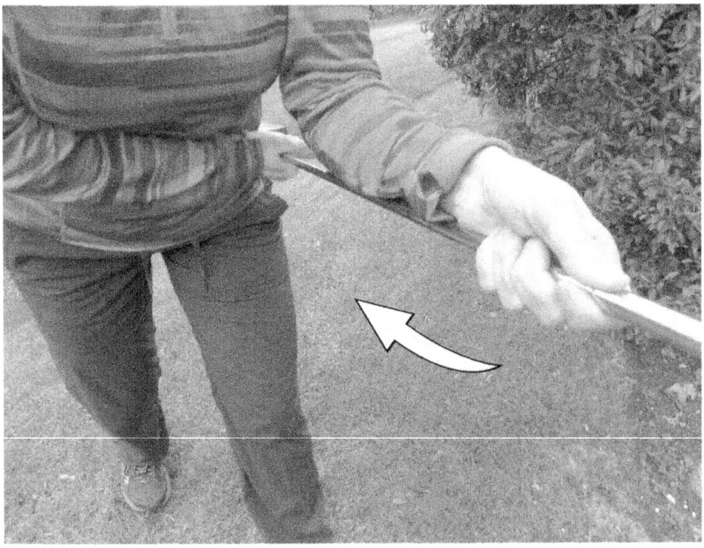

Chest – Chest Height Club Press Together

NOTE: The position for this exercise is virtually identical to that of the previous exercise, the Chest Height Club Pull-Apart. The important difference is that instead of pulling the club apart to perform an exercise targeting the rear upper back muscles, you press the club together to exercise the chest muscles.

Stand upright with your feet approximately shoulder-width apart. Hold the club in front of you at chest height and grip the club firmly. The hand position can vary according to your preference. It can range from close, where both hands touch, and wide, where the hands are wider than shoulder-width apart. Each position has merit and will exercise the muscles in a different position, so the choice is yours. Be sure to vary the hand position in each workout session you perform. In this position, apply pressure to push the club together and exercise the chest muscles.

The harder you engage the muscles, the more intense the exercise becomes, so always be sure to exercise at a level of force and intensity that best suits your ability.

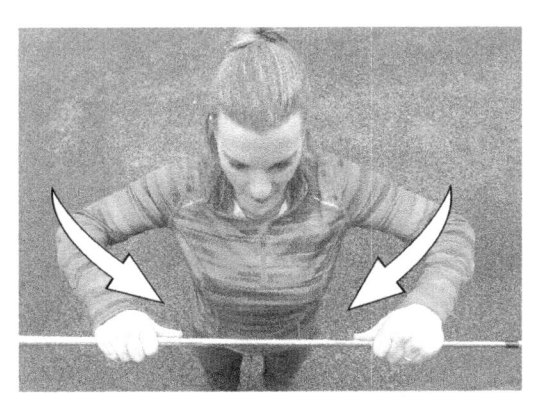

When you perform an isometric exercise, never hold your breath. Always breathe deeply and naturally, which will be about 10 full breaths in and out at a rate of about 1 second per full breath. Perform each exercise for no less than 7 seconds and no longer than 10.

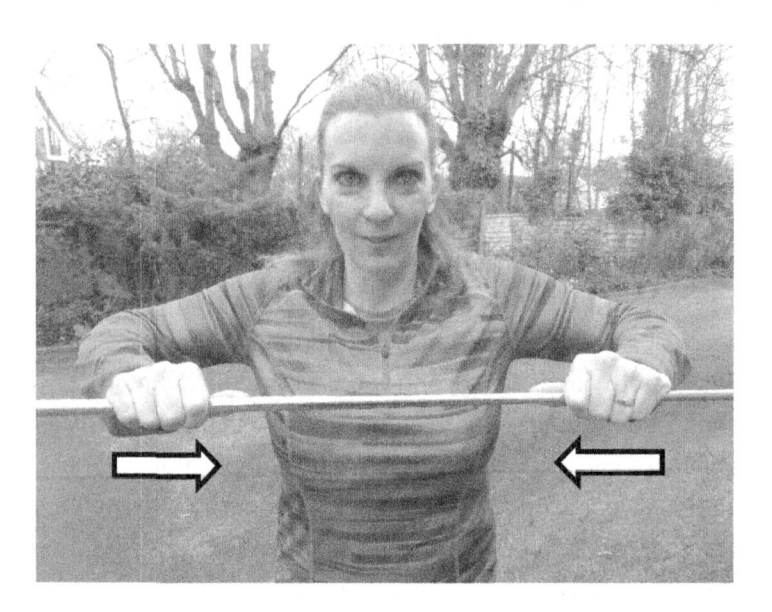

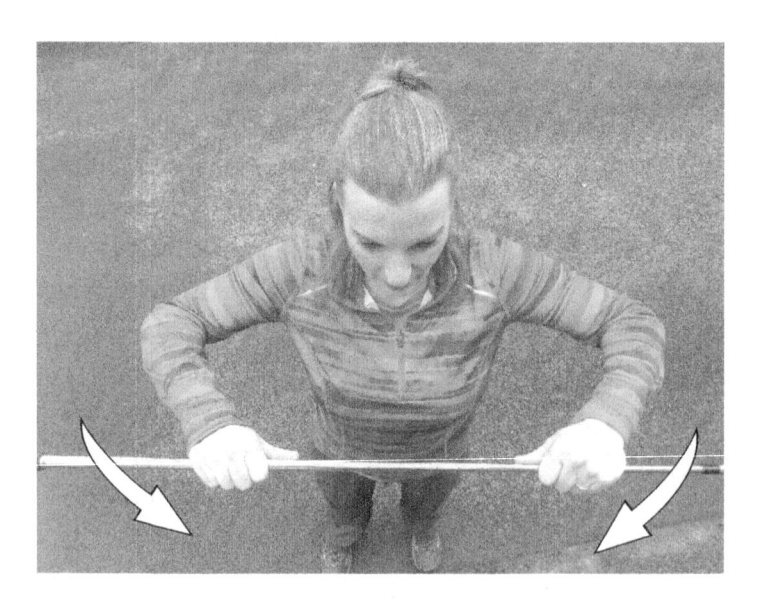

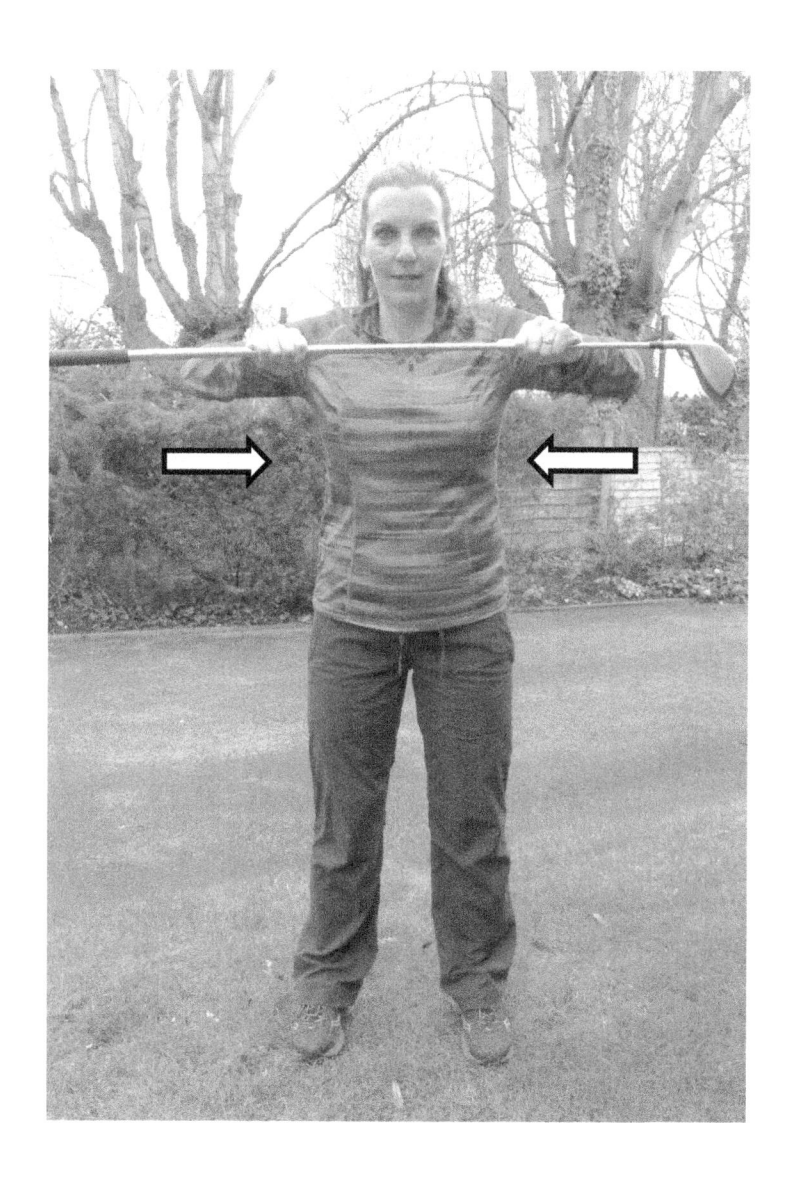

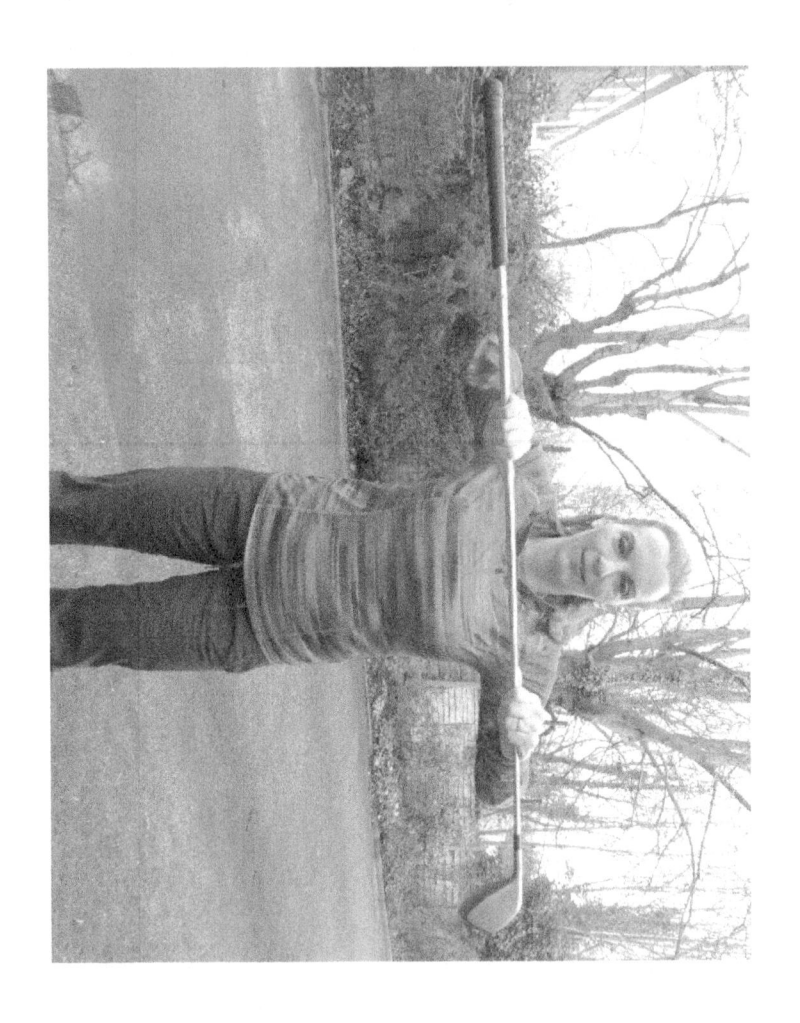

Legs – Calf Double Heel Raise

Stand upright with your feet approximately shoulder-width apart. Hold the club upright in front of you with the tip on solid ground. Hold the club with both hands for balance. Two clubs can be used if you wish. However, increased core stability benefits are gained if only a single club is used. In this position, raise both heels off the floor as far as possible to tense and engage the calf muscles of the lower legs. Be sure to exercise both sides of the body.

The harder you engage the muscles, the more intense the exercise becomes, so always be sure to exercise at a level of force and intensity that best suits your ability.

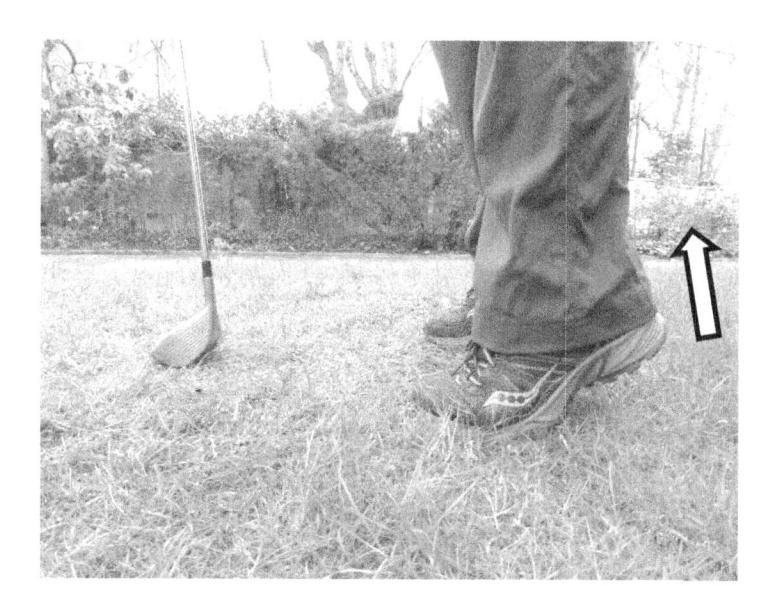

When you perform an isometric exercise, never hold your breath. Always breathe deeply and naturally, which will be about 10 full breaths in and out at a rate of about 1 second per full breath. Perform each exercise for no less than 7 seconds and no longer than 10.

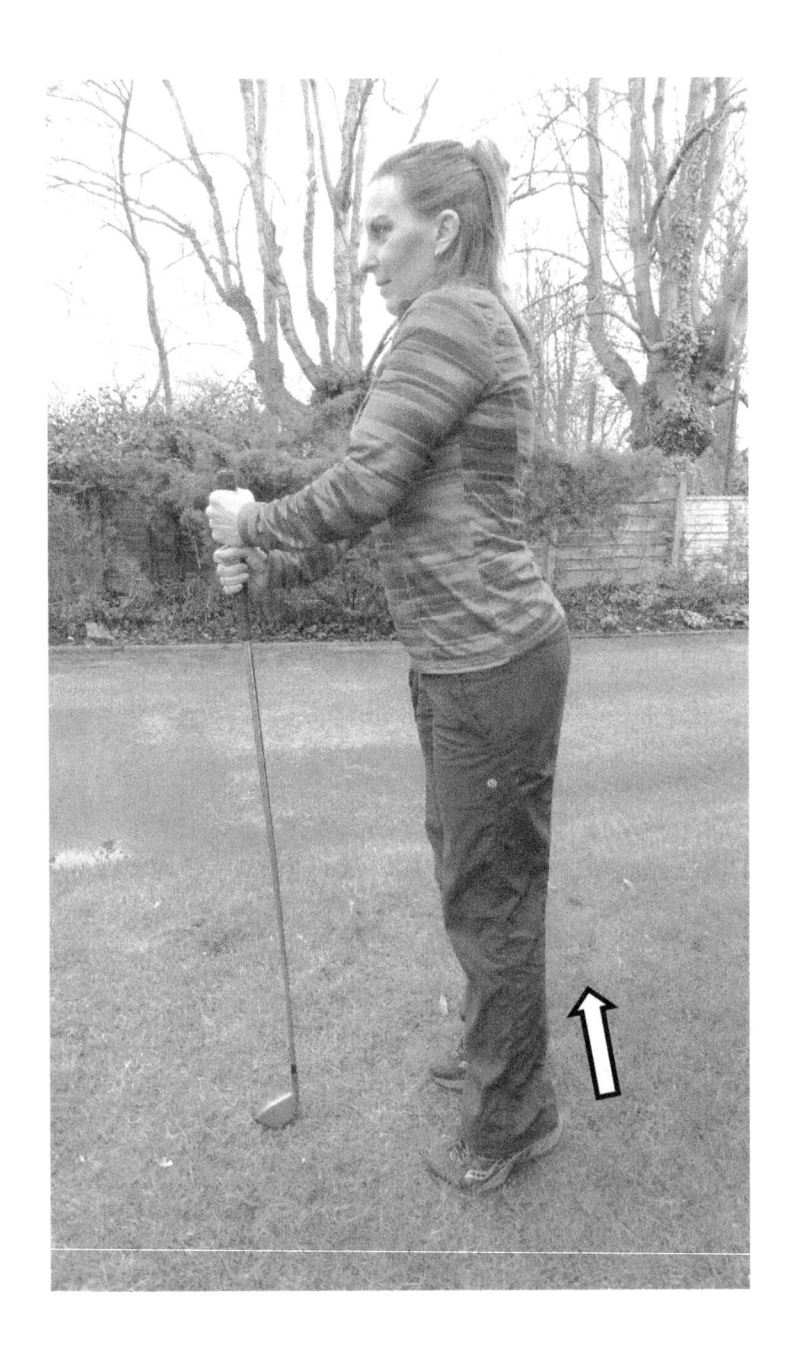

Legs – Calf Single Heel Raise

Stand upright with your feet approximately shoulder-width apart. Hold the club upright in front of you with the tip on solid ground. Hold the club with both hands for balance. Two clubs can be used if you wish. However, increased core stability benefits are gained if only a single club is used. In this position, raise one heel off the floor as far as possible to tense and engage the calf muscles of the lower legs. Tuck the raised foot of the other leg on or around the calf of the leg you are exercising.

The harder you engage the muscles, the more intense the exercise becomes, so always be sure to exercise at a level of force and intensity that best suits your ability. When you perform an isometric exercise, never hold your breath. Always breathe deeply and naturally, which will be about 10 full breaths in and out at a rate of about 1 second per full breath. Perform each exercise for no less than 7 seconds and no longer than 10. Be sure to exercise both sides of the body.

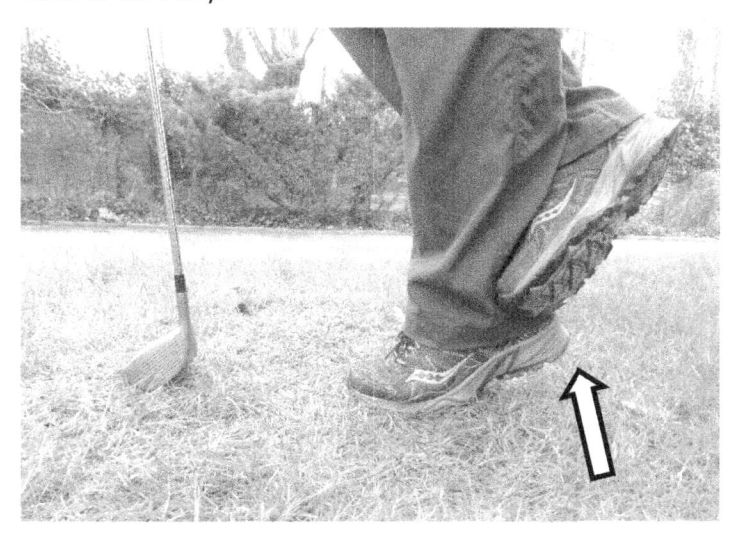

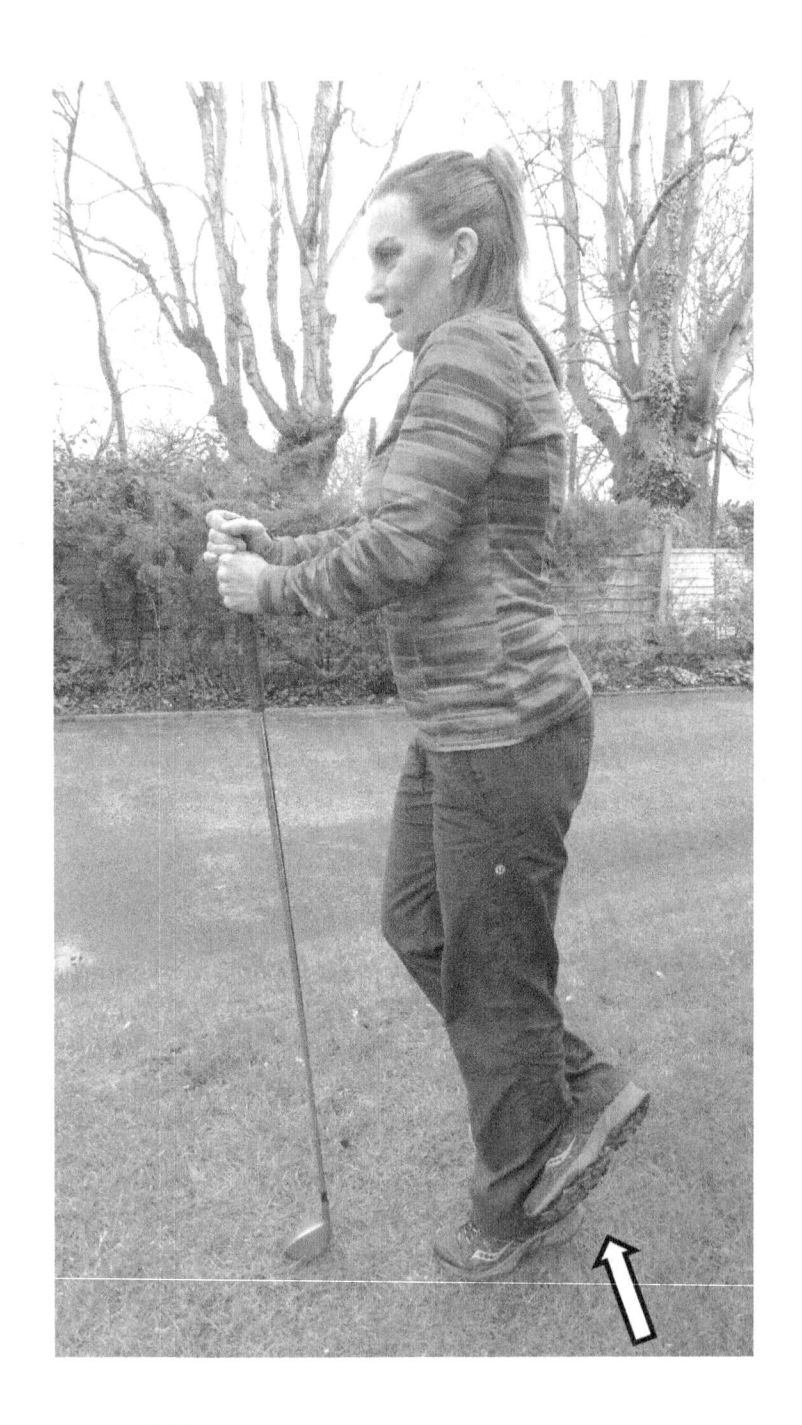

Legs – Calf Immovable Object Single Heel Raise

Stand upright with your feet approximately shoulder-width apart. Select a safe, immovable object that you can push against. This can be a vehicle, a tree, a fence, a wall, or a rock, etc. The immovable object will provide a more intense and challenging exercise resistance than bodyweight alone. In this position, raise one heel off the floor as far as possible to tense and engage the calf muscles of the lower legs as you push to attempt to move the object using your calf muscles as the driving force. Tuck the raised foot of the other leg on, or around the calf of the leg you are exercising. The harder you engage the muscles, the more intense the exercise becomes, so always be sure to exercise at a level of force and intensity that best suits your ability. When you perform an isometric exercise, never hold your breath. Always breathe deeply and naturally, which will be about 10 full breaths in and out at a rate of about 1 second per full breath. Perform each exercise for no less than 7 seconds and no longer than 10. Be sure to exercise both sides of the body.

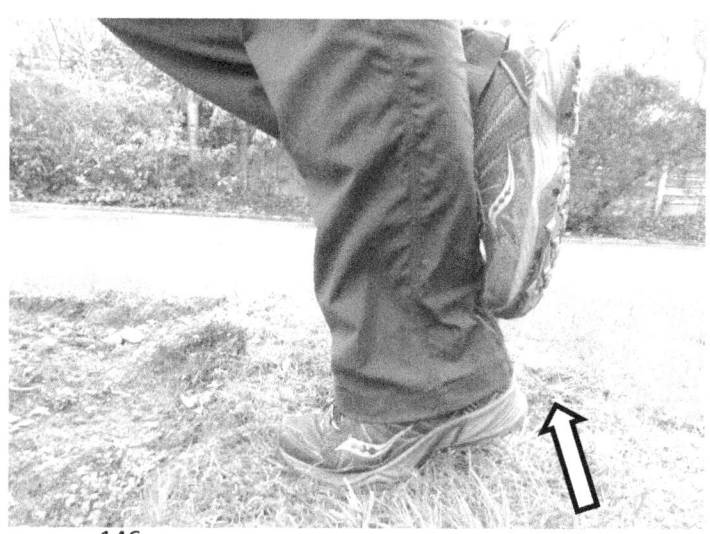

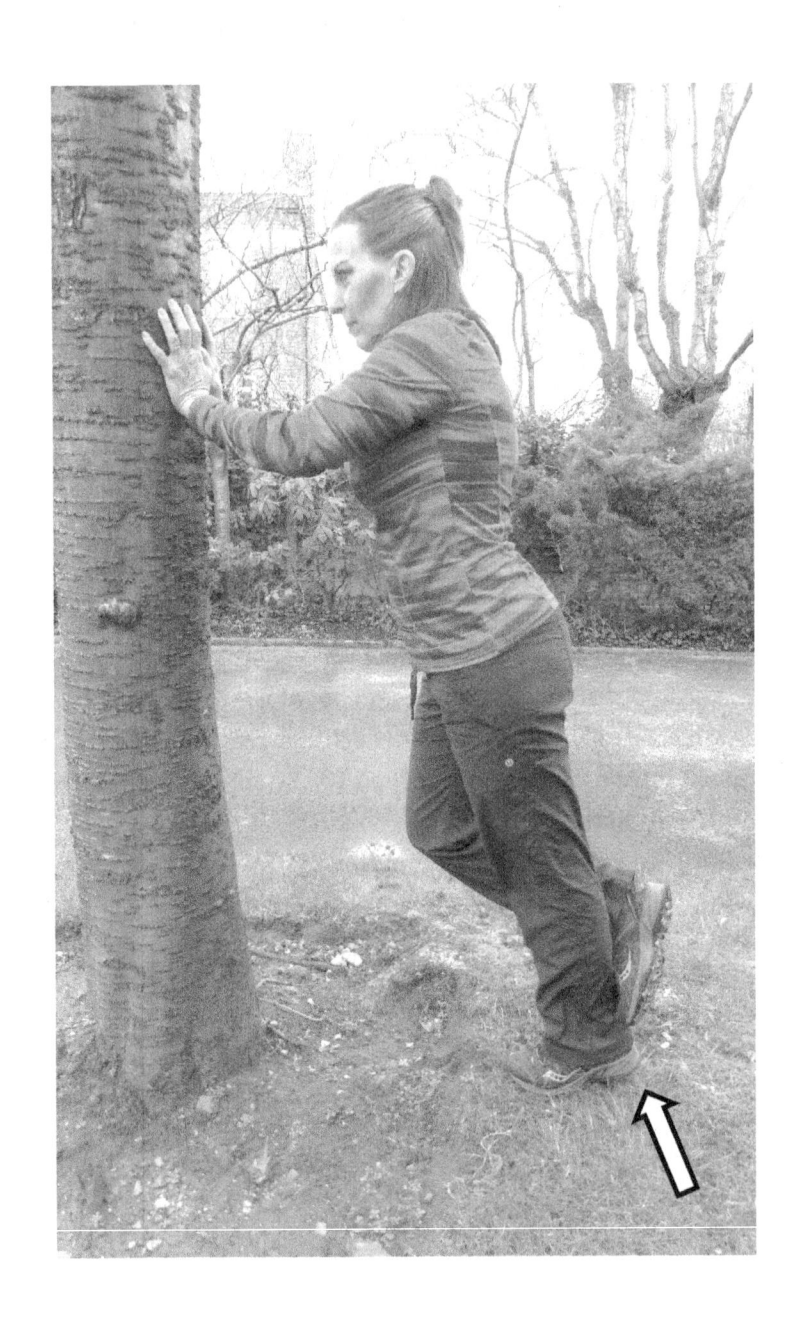

Legs – Thigh Lunge Club-Assisted

Stand upright with your feet approximately shoulder-width apart. Step straight forward with one leg and bend the knee carefully and gently until your upper thigh is approximately parallel to the floor. For balance, keep your hands forward and hold either a club, a tree, or a fence, etc. Hold the bent-knee lunge position to exercise the front upper thigh and the buttocks. Be sure to exercise both sides of the body.

The harder you engage the muscles, the more intense the exercise becomes, so always be sure to exercise at a level of force and intensity that best suits your ability.

When you perform an isometric exercise, never hold your breath. Always breathe deeply and naturally, which will be about 10 full breaths in and out at a rate of about 1 second per full breath. Perform each exercise for no less than 7 seconds and no longer than 10.

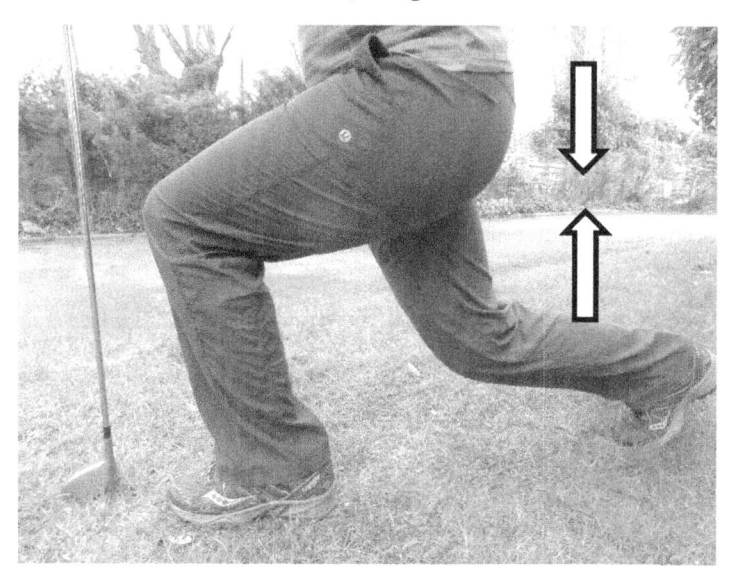

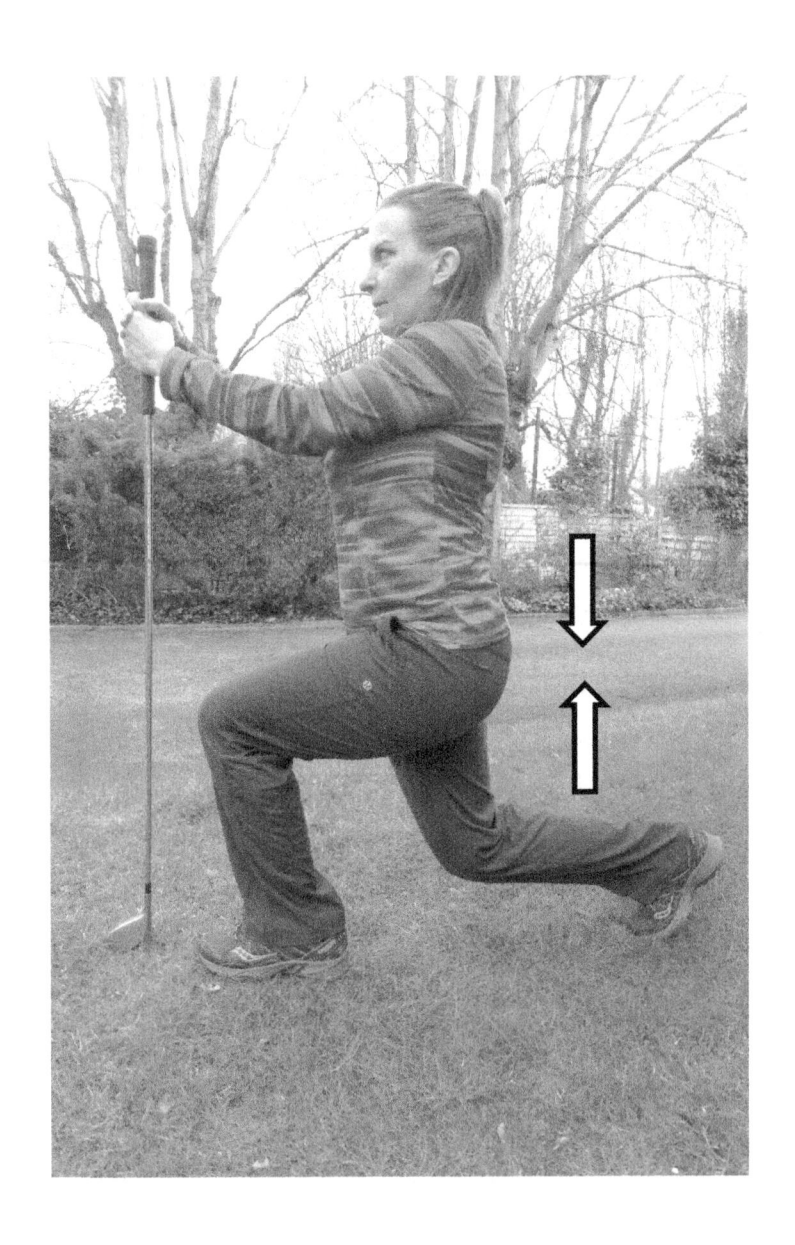

Legs – Thigh Lunge Advanced Club-Balanced

This exercise is almost the same as the previous one, which uses the golf club to aid your balance. In this more advanced variation, the golf club is not used as an aid to balance by keeping it touching the ground. Instead, the golf club is held horizontally in outstretched arms to aid your balance, similar to a tightrope walker's pole. Step straight forward with one leg and bend the knee carefully until your upper thigh is approximately parallel to the floor. Hold the bent-knee lunge position to exercise the front upper thigh and the buttocks. Be sure to exercise both sides of the body. The harder you engage the muscles, the more intense the exercise becomes, so always be sure to exercise at a level of force and intensity that best suits your ability. When you perform an isometric exercise, never hold your breath. Always breathe deeply and naturally, which will be about 10 full breaths in and out at a rate of about 1 second per full breath. Perform each exercise for no less than 7 seconds and no longer than 10.

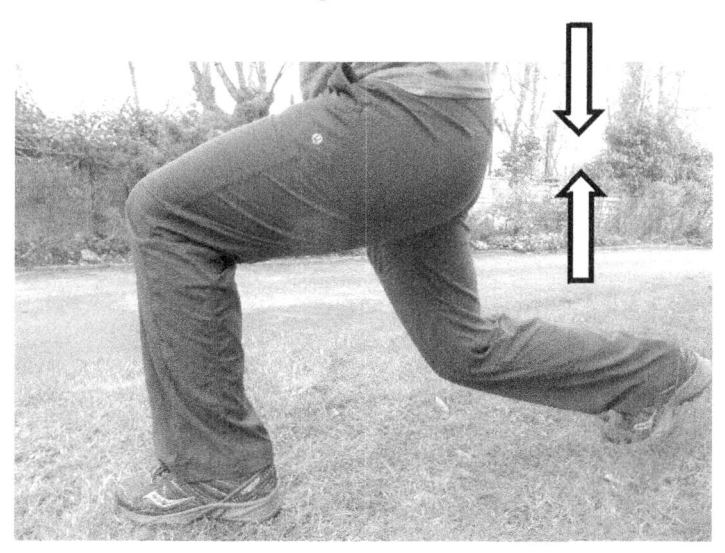

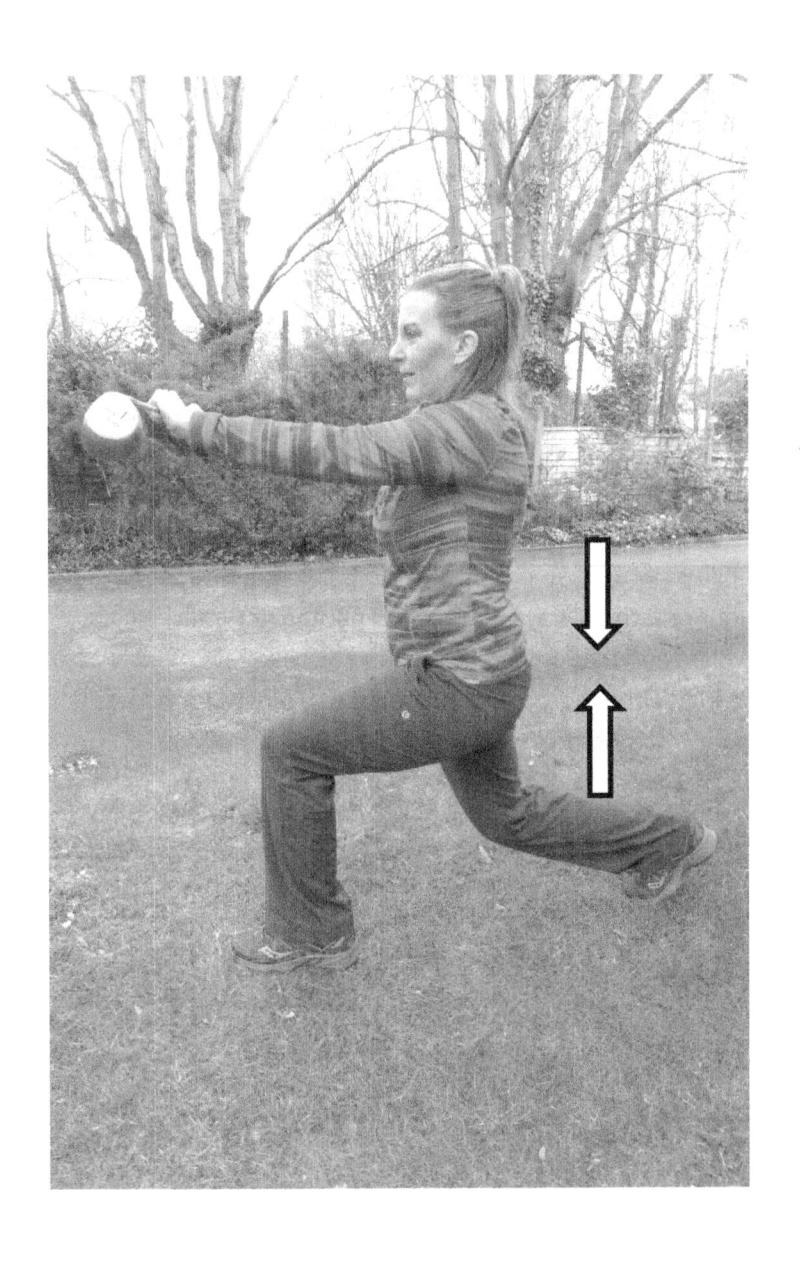

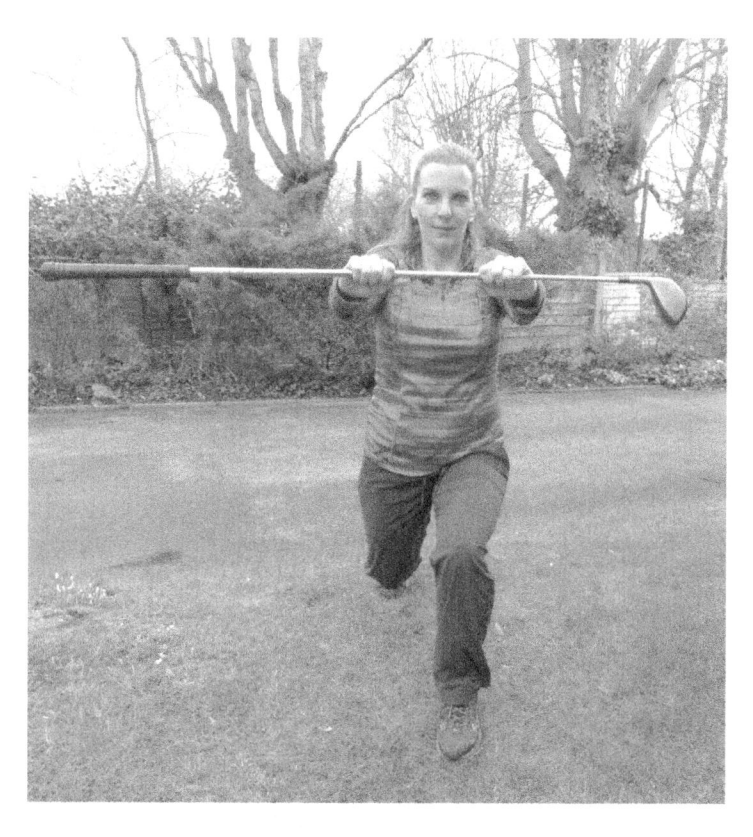

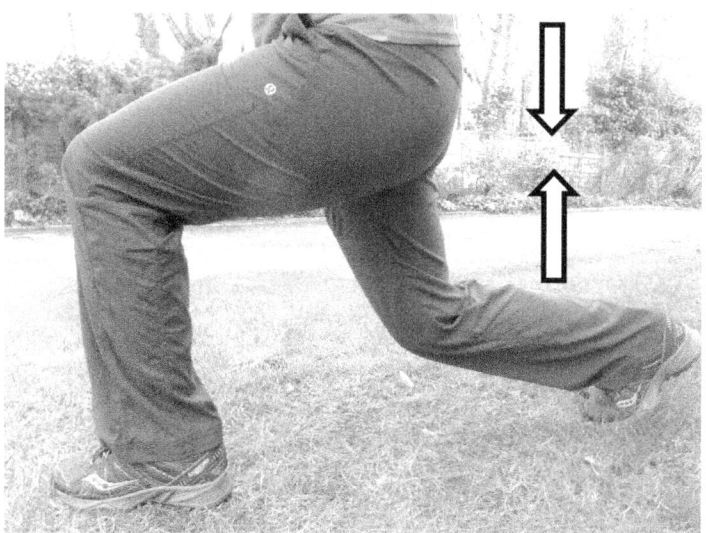

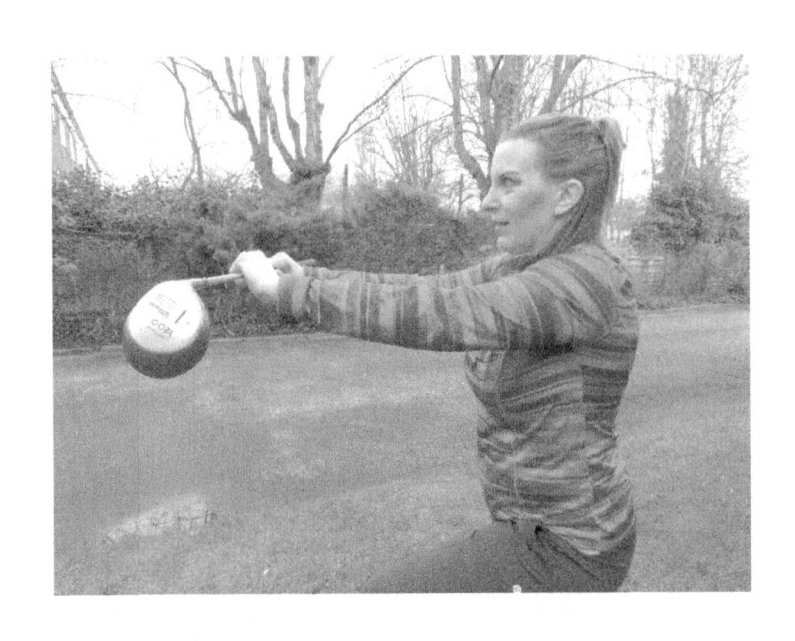

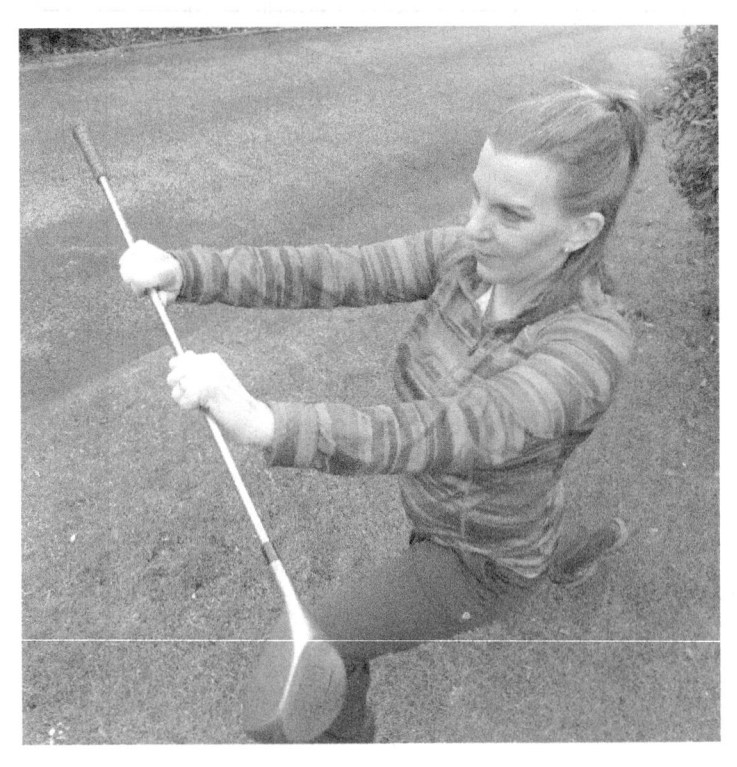

Legs – Thigh Squat Club in Front

Stand upright with your feet approximately shoulder-width apart. Place a club in front of you on solid ground and hold it to aid your balance. Keeping your back straight and bending forward slightly only from the hips, bend the knees to assume a squat position. This will exercise the front upper thighs and buttocks. The deeper the squat position, the more intense the exercise becomes.

The harder you engage the muscles, the more intense the exercise becomes, so always be sure to exercise at a level of force and intensity that best suits your ability. When you perform an isometric exercise, never hold your breath. Always breathe deeply and naturally, which will be about 10 full breaths in and out at a rate of about 1 second per full breath. Perform each exercise for no less than 7 seconds and no longer than 10.

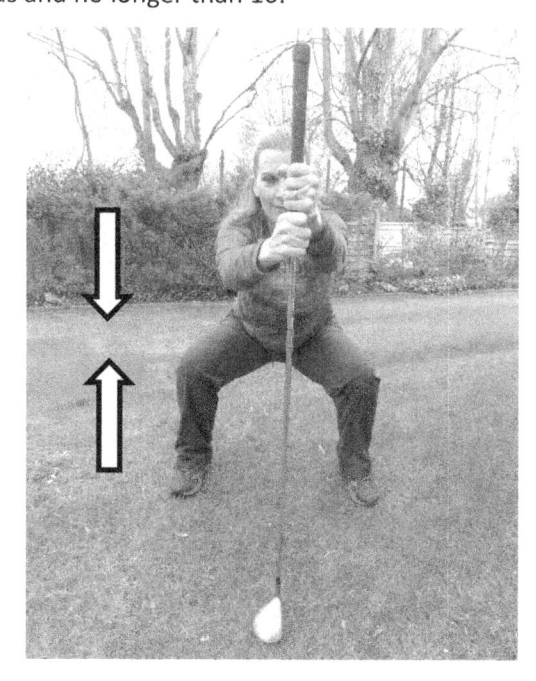

155

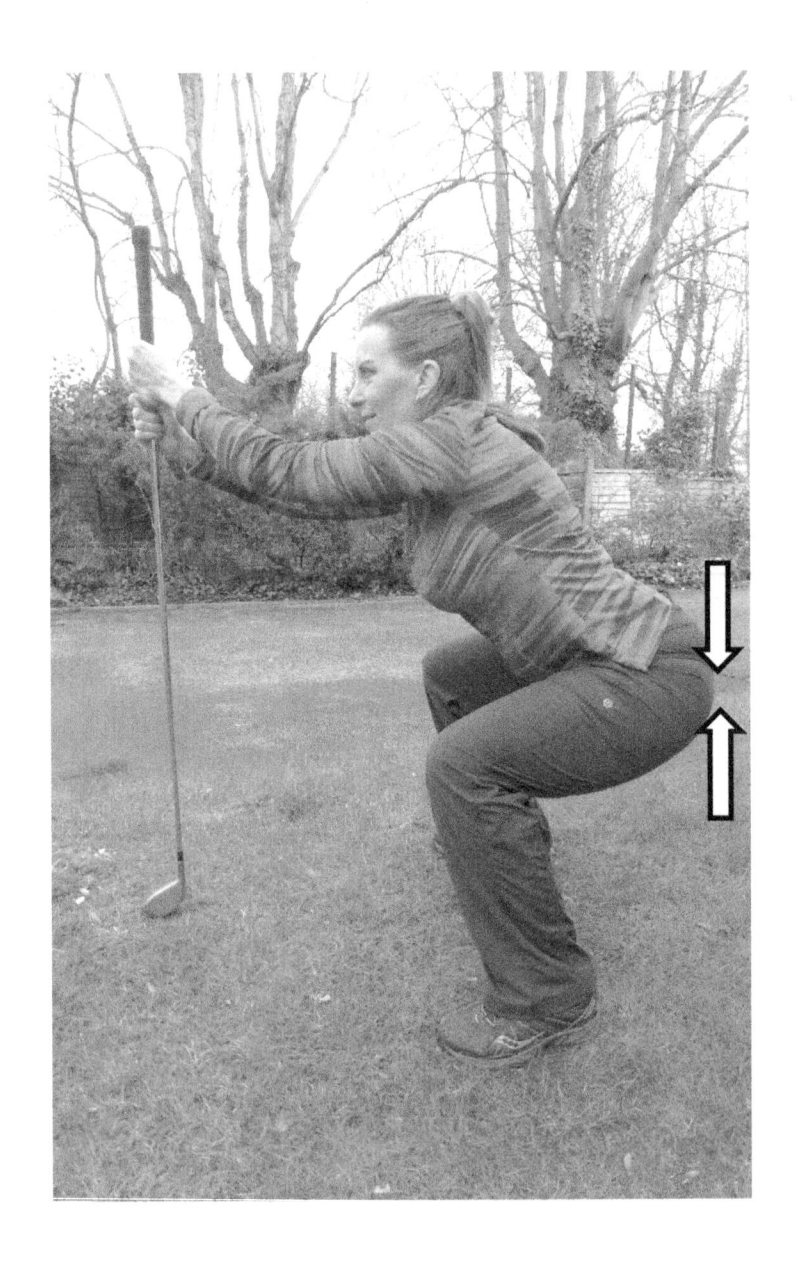

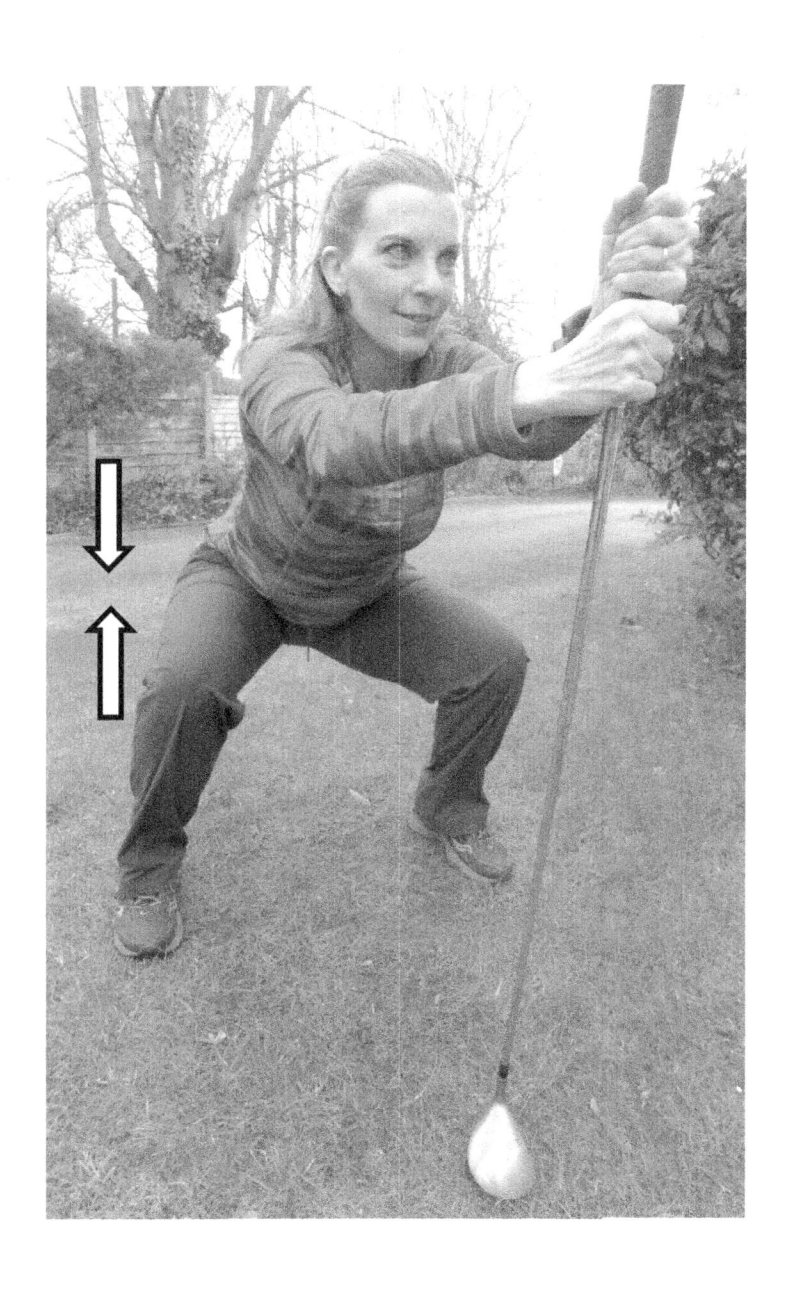

Legs – Thigh Squat Club Across Back

Stand upright with your feet approximately shoulder-width apart. Place a club evenly across your shoulders behind your neck. Keeping your back straight and bending forward slightly only from the hips, bend the knees to assume a squat position. This will exercise the front upper thighs and buttocks. The deeper the squat position, the more intense the exercise becomes. This exercise is much more challenging than when performed by holding the club on the ground in front of you. The harder you engage the muscles, the more intense the exercise becomes, so always be sure to exercise at a level of force that best suits your ability. When you perform an isometric exercise, never hold your breath. Always breathe deeply and naturally, which will be about 10 full breaths in and out at a rate of about 1 second per full breath. Perform each exercise for no less than 7 seconds and no longer than 10.

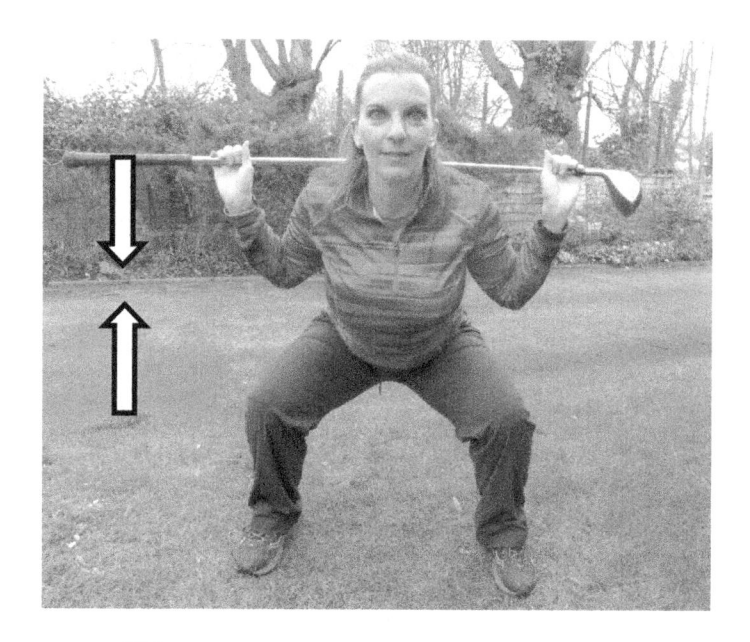

159

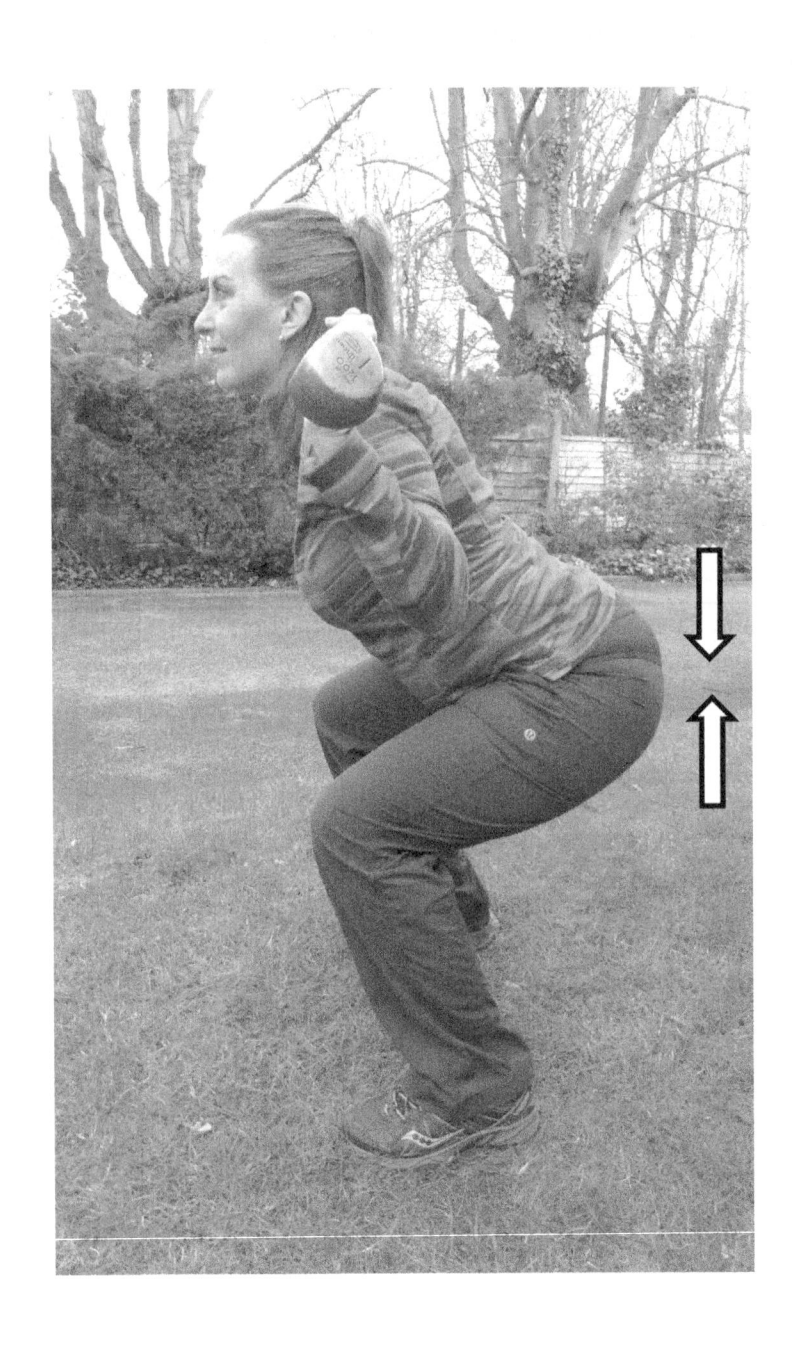

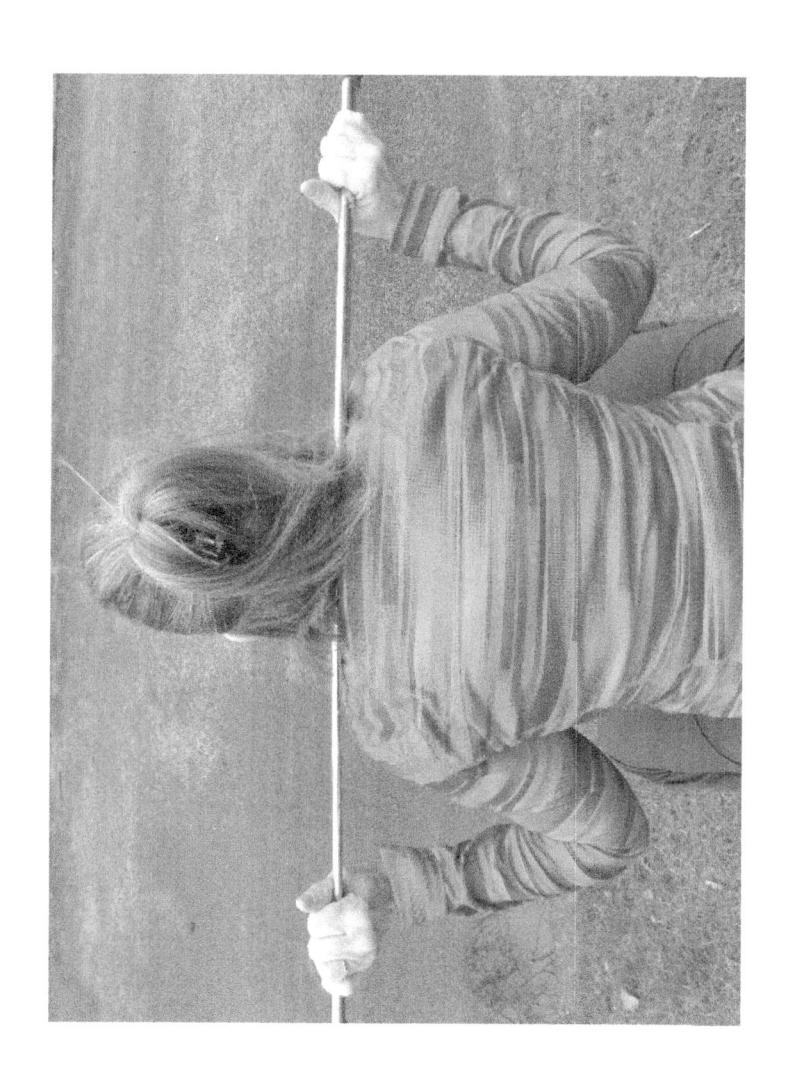

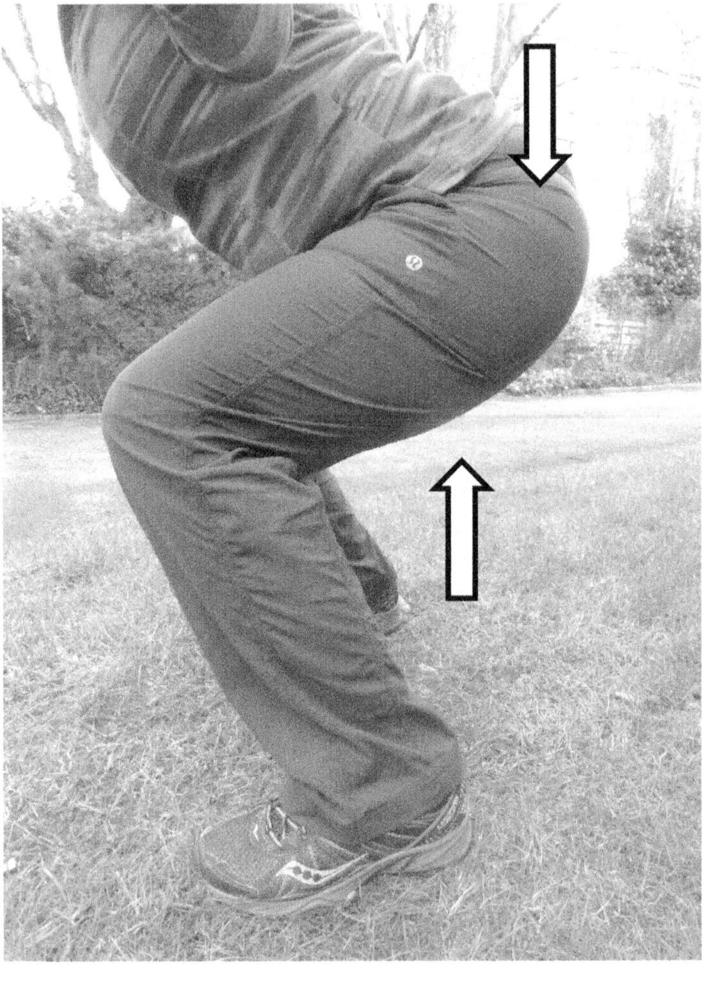

Shoulders – Club Press Above Head

Stand upright with your feet approximately shoulder-width apart. Hold a club above your head with your hands slightly wider than shoulder-width apart. In this position, apply force to press both inwards and slightly upwards at the same time. This will target your entire shoulder, upper back, and neck region. The harder you engage the muscles, the more intense the exercise becomes, so always be sure to exercise at a level of force and intensity that best suits your ability. When you perform an isometric exercise, never hold your breath. Always breathe deeply and naturally, which will be about 10 full breaths in and out at a rate of about 1 second per full breath. Perform each exercise for no less than 7 seconds and no longer than 10. NOTE: The exercise can be performed with the club as shown or in a position just behind your head. However, both positions have merit, so mix them up and perform different positions in each workout you perform.

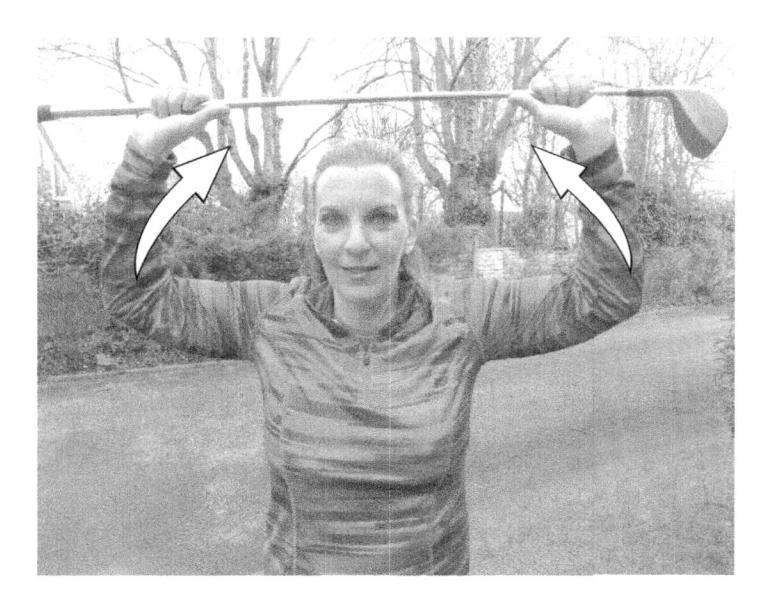

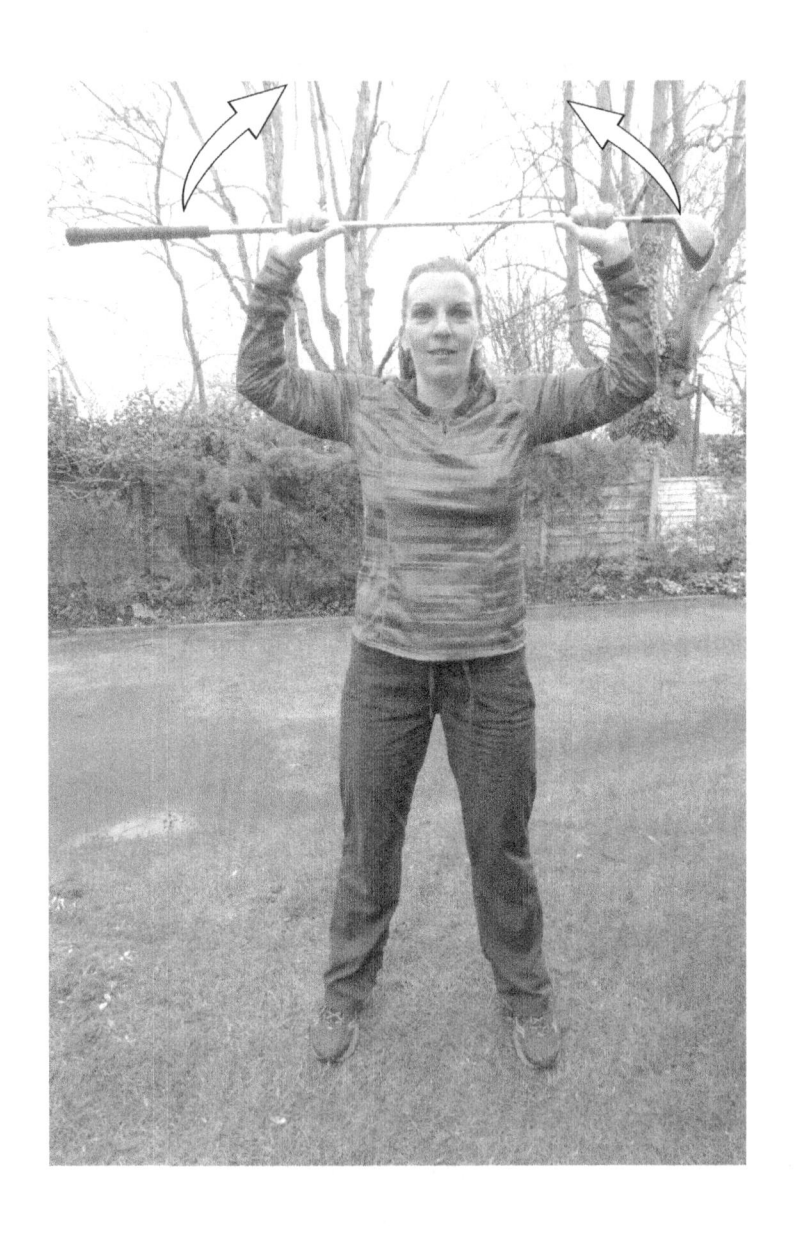

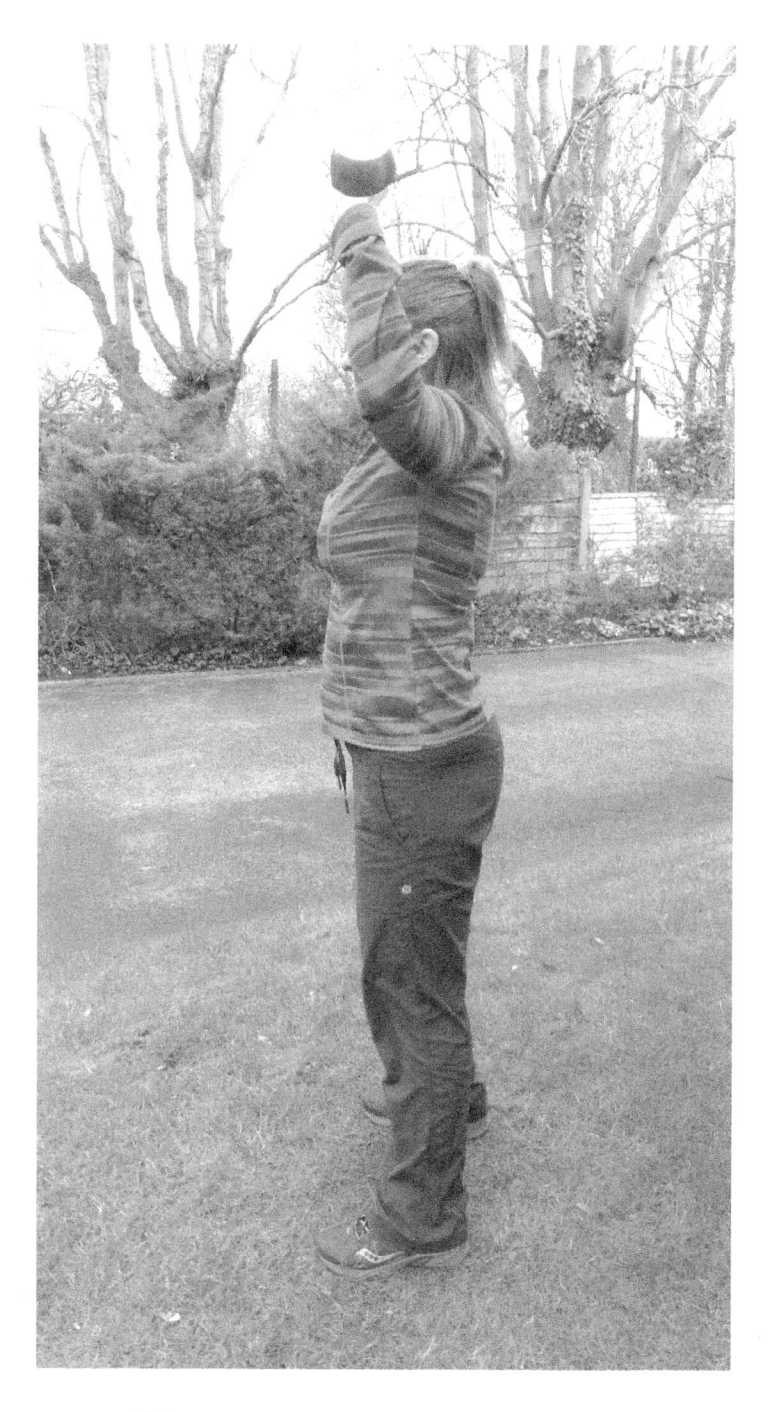

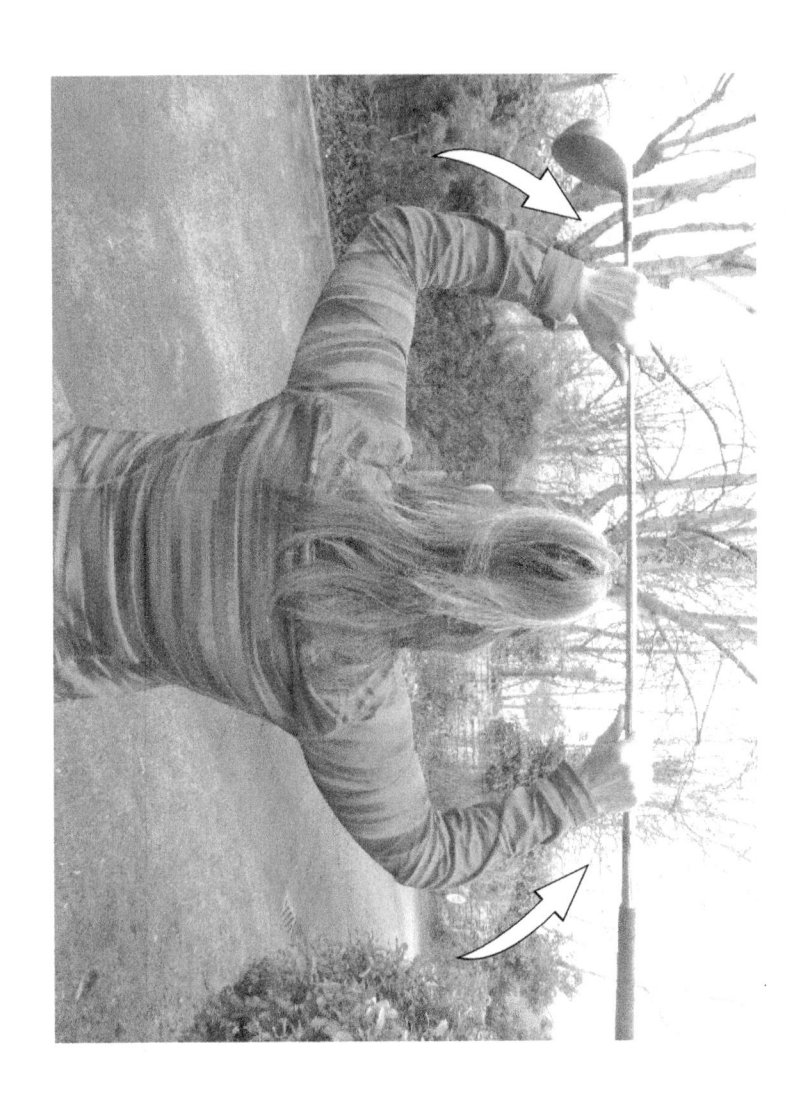

Shoulders – Club Side Lateral Raise

Stand upright with your feet approximately shoulder-width apart. Hold a club in both hands in front of you, raised slightly to one side. The leading arm to that side should be locked in a slightly bent position so the hand's little finger is pointing sideways. Apply resistance with the leading arm to try and raise the club sideways while it is resisted from moving by the other hand. This will target the shoulder muscles of both the leading and lower securing arm. Be sure to exercise both sides of the body.

The harder you engage the muscles, the more intense the exercise becomes, so always be sure to exercise at a level of force and intensity that best suits your ability. When you perform an isometric exercise, never hold your breath. Always breathe deeply and naturally, which will be about 10 full breaths in and out at a rate of about 1 second per full breath. Perform each exercise for no less than 7 seconds and no longer than 10.

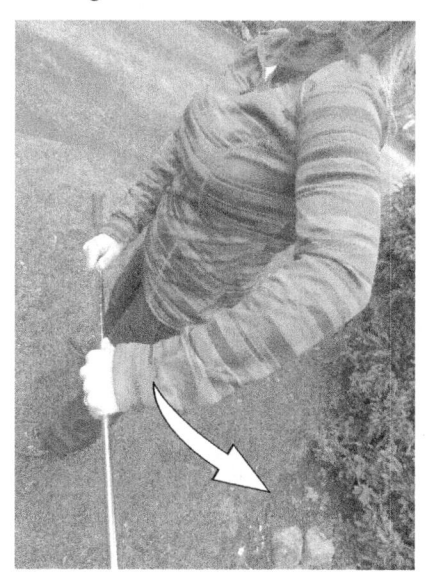

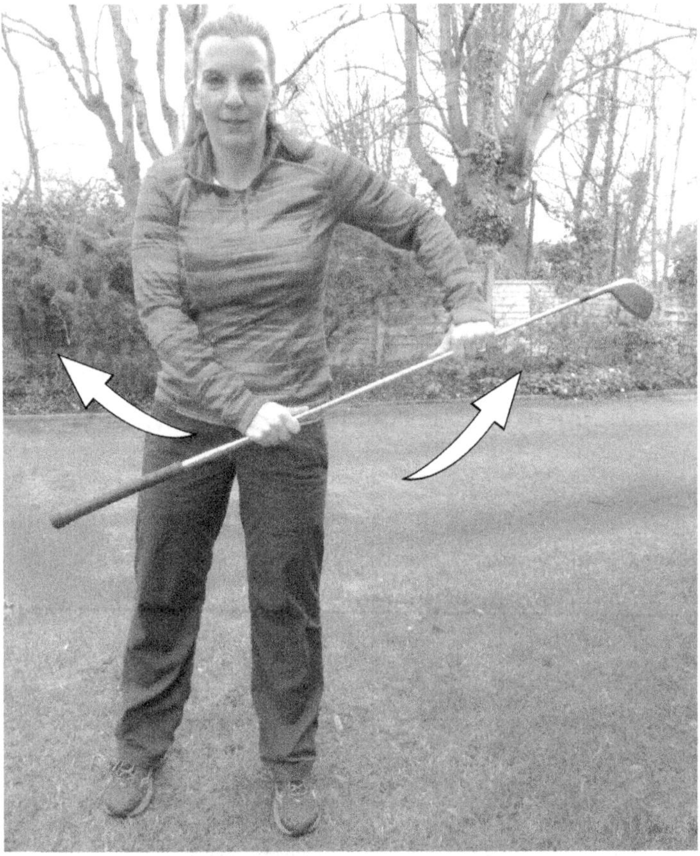

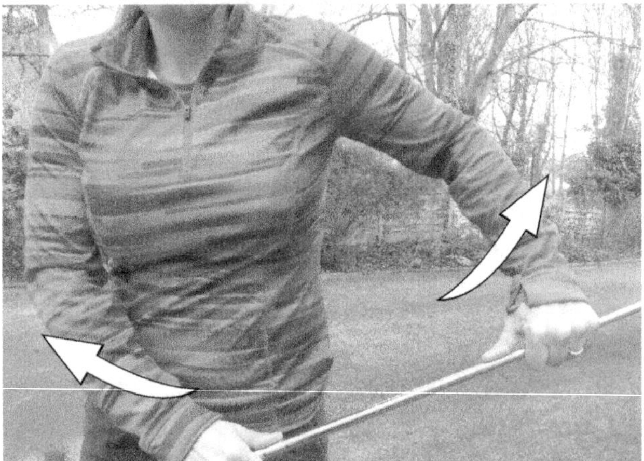

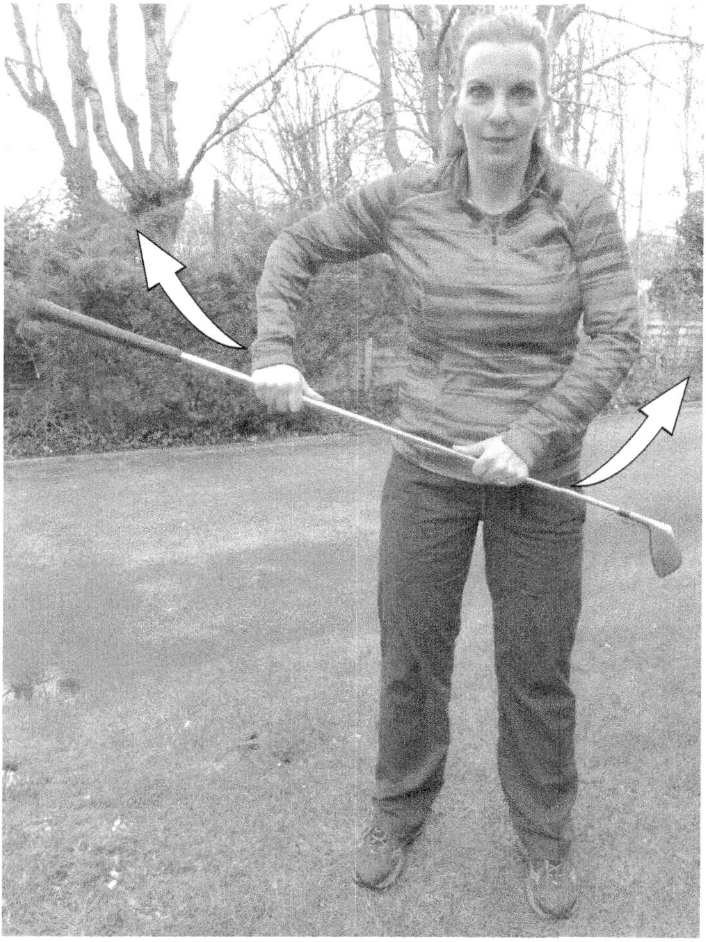

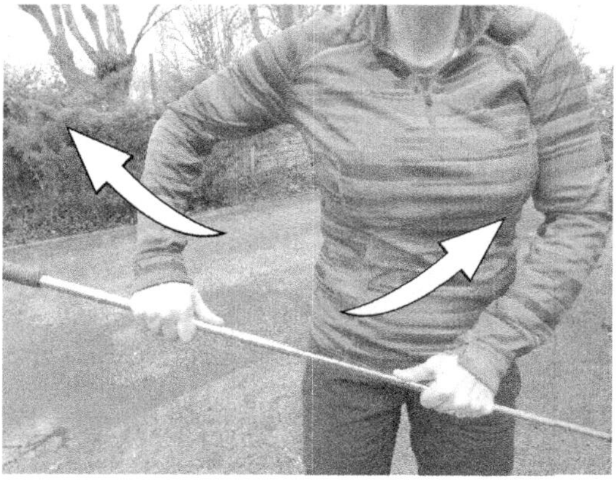

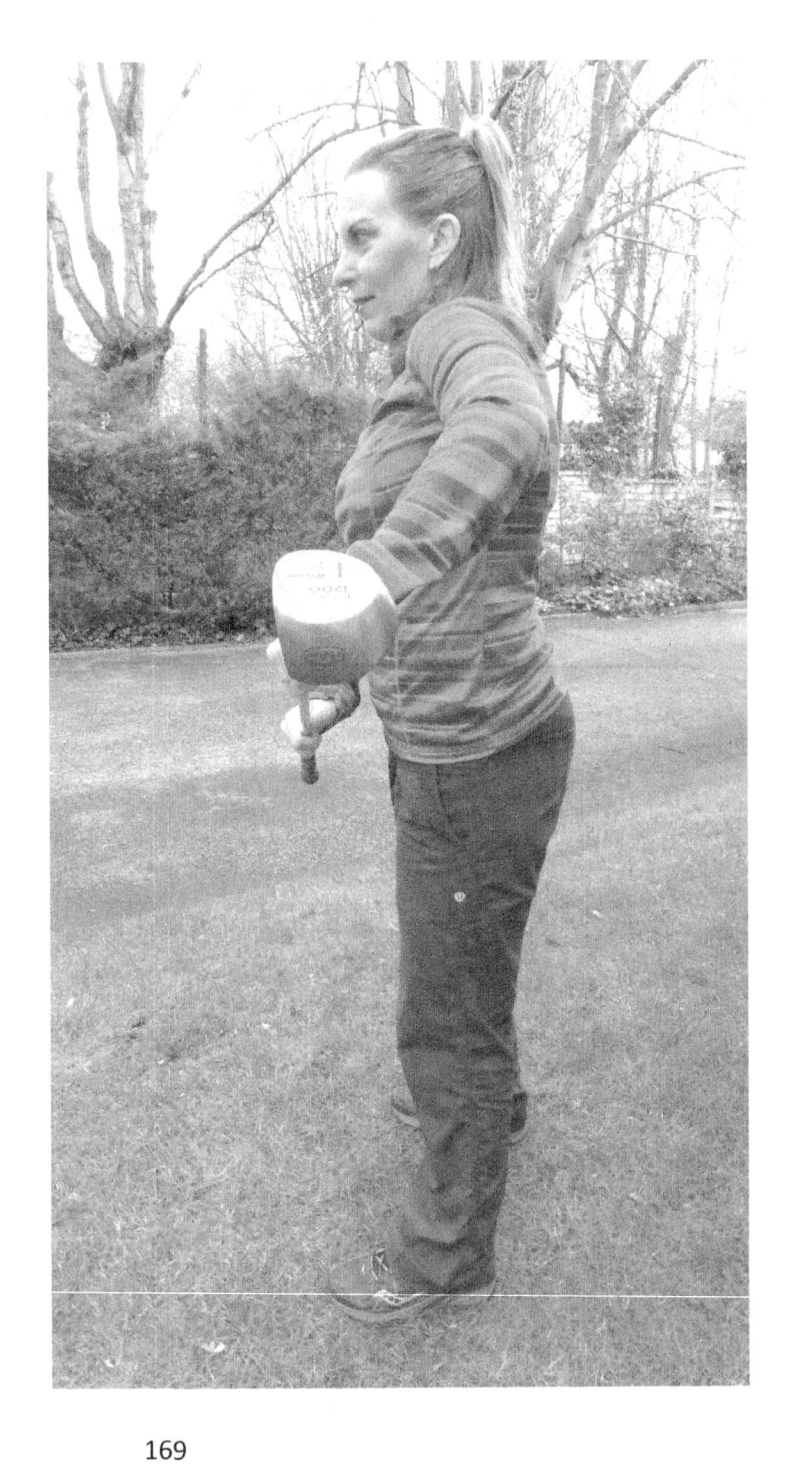

Shoulders – Club Mid-Point Lateral Raise

Stand upright with your feet approximately shoulder-width apart. Hold a club in both hands in front of you at the mid-point of the body at approximately waist height. Both arms should be locked in a slightly bent position so the little finger of each hand is pointing sideways. Apply equal resistance with both arms to try and raise the club sideways and upwards while it is resisted from moving by the other hand. This will target the shoulder muscles of both the leading and lower securing arm. Be sure to exercise both sides of the body. The harder you engage the muscles, the more intense the exercise becomes, so always be sure to exercise at a level of force that best suits your ability. When you perform an isometric exercise, never hold your breath. Always breathe deeply and naturally, which will be about 10 full breaths in and out at a rate of about 1 second per full breath. Perform each exercise for no less than 7 seconds and no longer than 10.

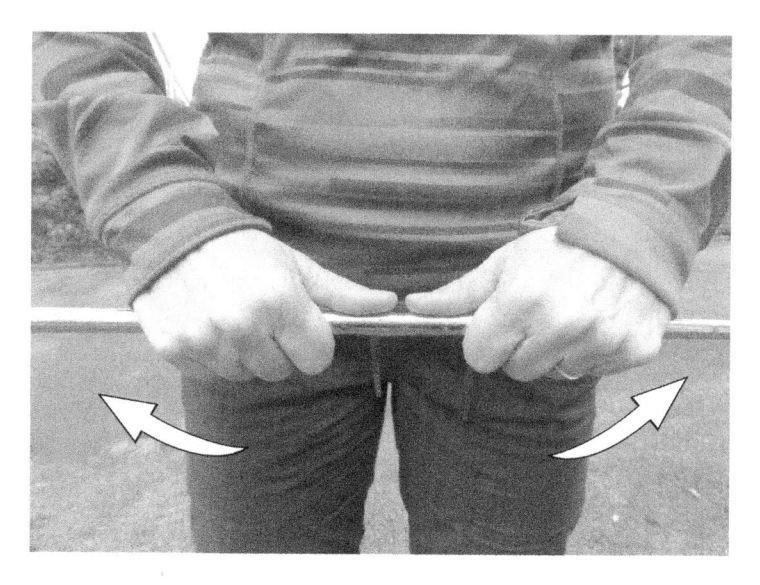

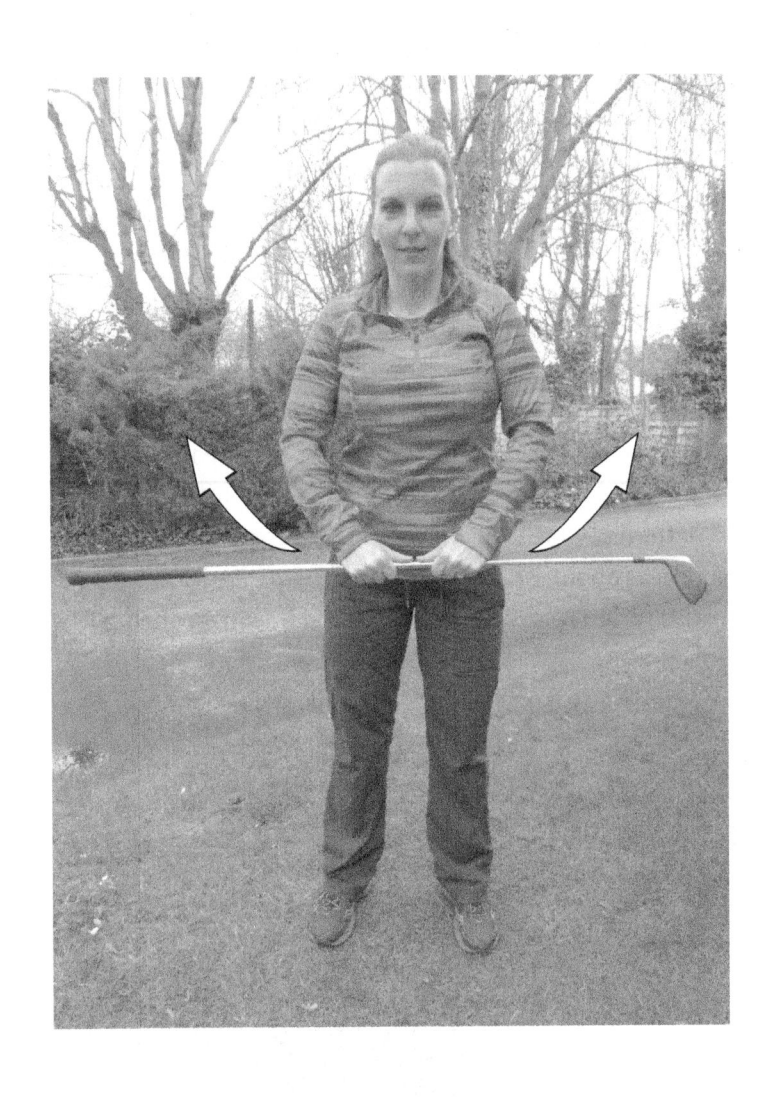

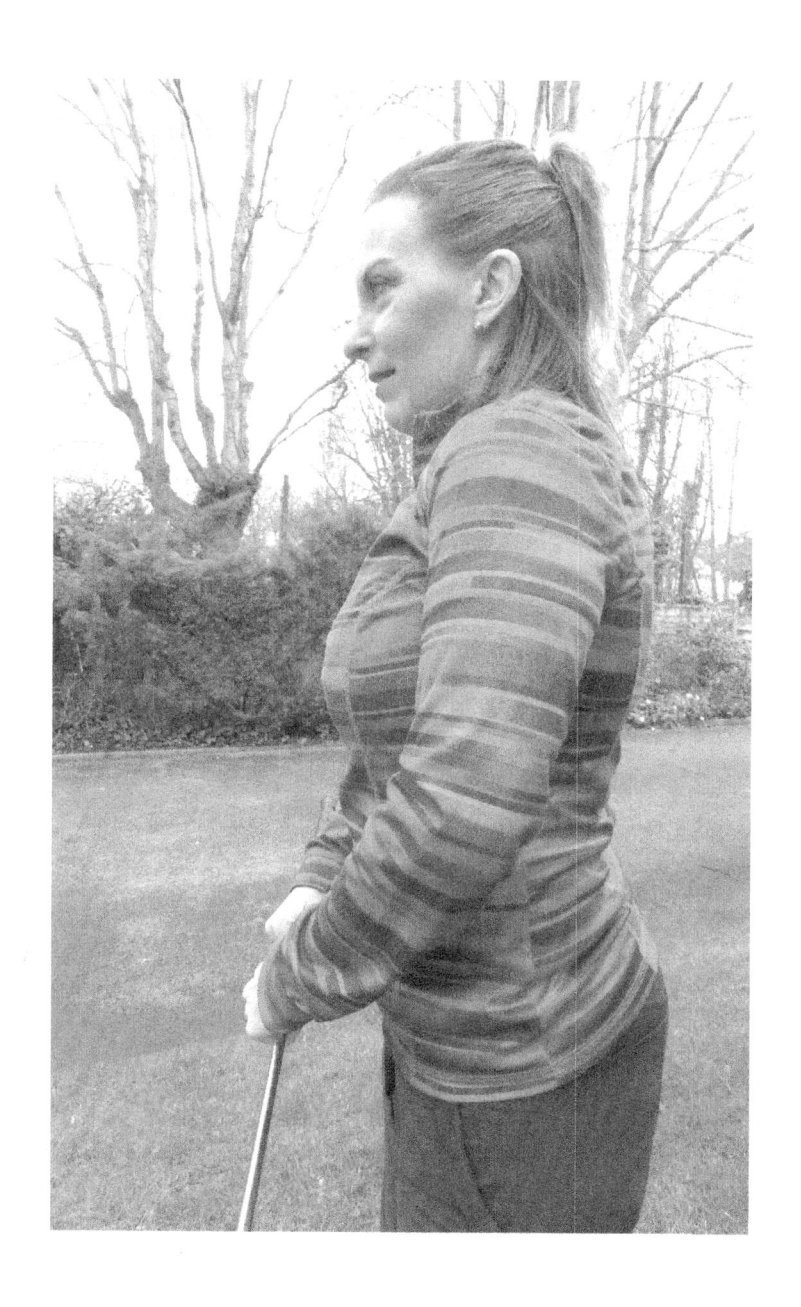

Shoulders – Club Front Raise

Stand upright with your feet approximately shoulder-width apart. Hold a club in both hands in front of you with one hand/arm higher than the other. Keep the higher hand/arm slightly bent and locked in that position. Apply resistance with the higher leading arm/hand to try and raise the club upwards directly in front of you while the other lower hand resists moving. This will target the shoulder muscles of the leading arm. Be sure to exercise both sides of the body.

The harder you engage the muscles, the more intense the exercise becomes, so always be sure to exercise at a level of force and intensity that best suits your ability. When you perform an isometric exercise, never hold your breath. Always breathe deeply and naturally, which will be about 10 full breaths in and out at a rate of about 1 second per full breath. Perform each exercise for no less than 7 seconds and no longer than 10.

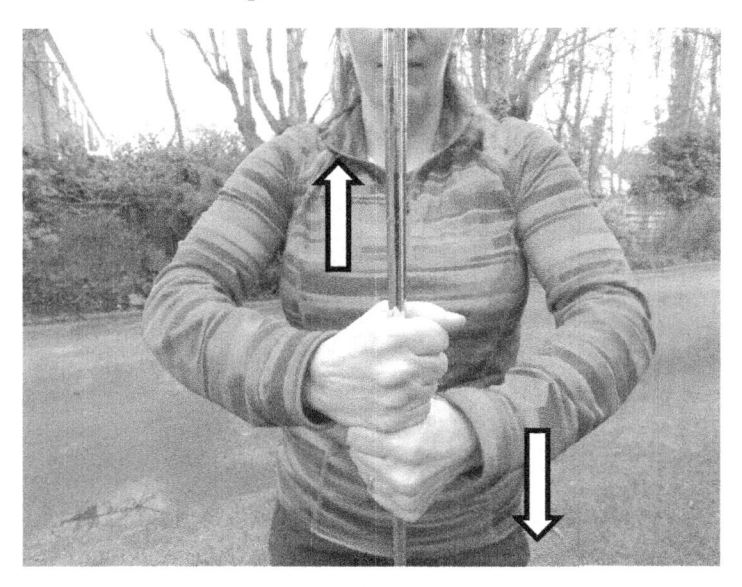

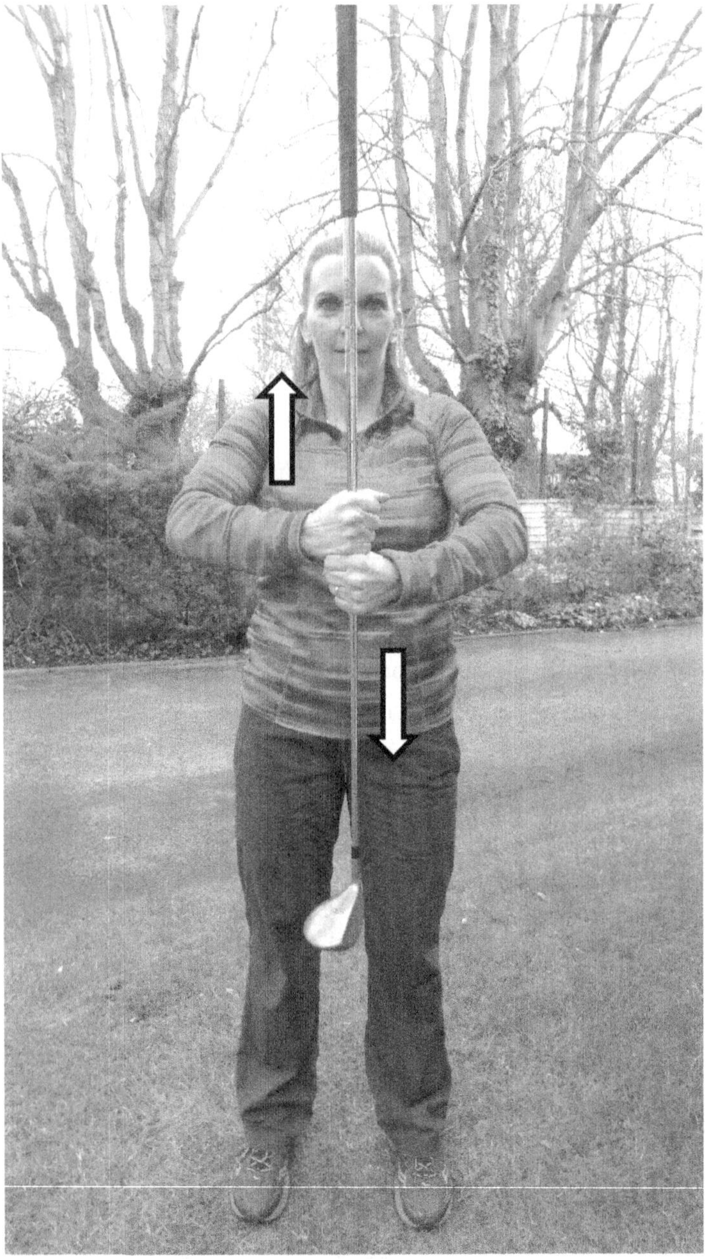

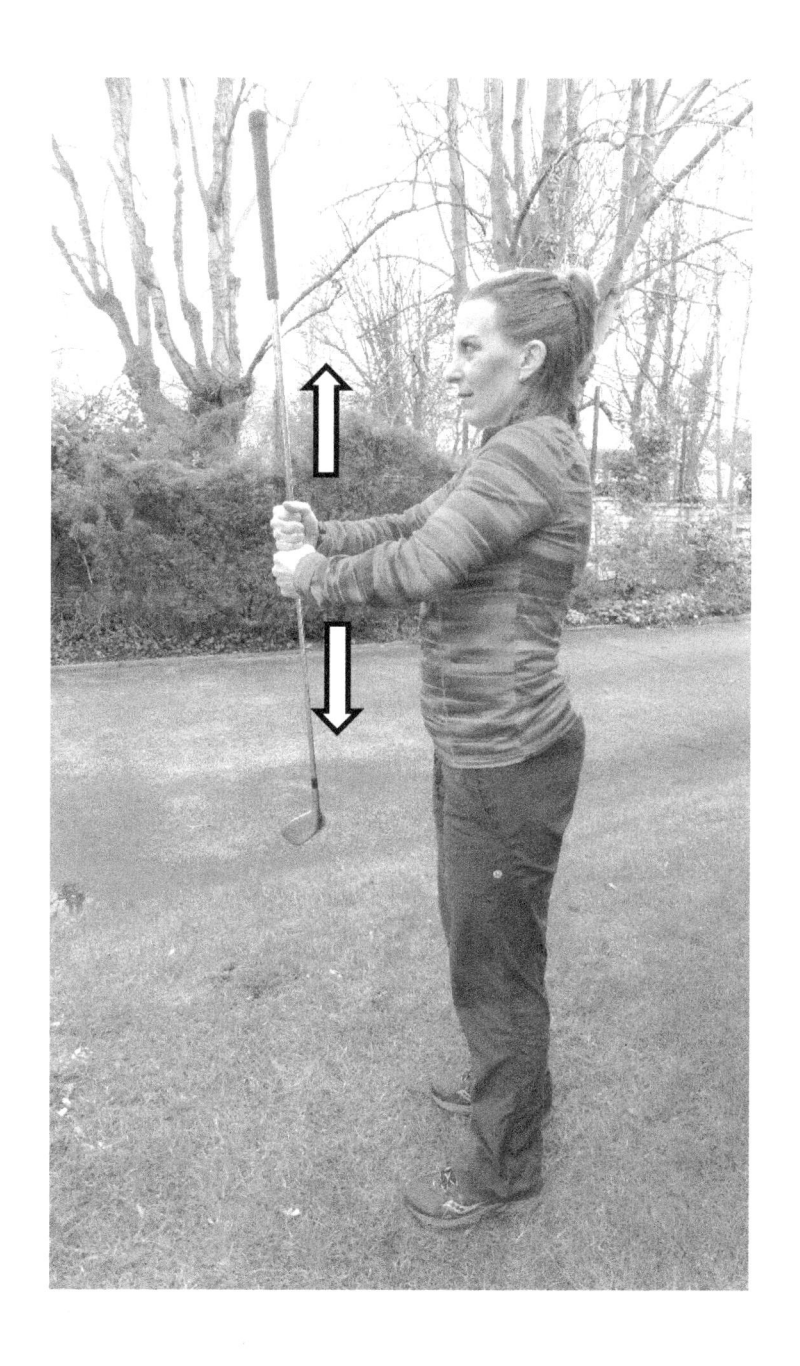

Golf Swing Door Pull
The Pre-Swing Pull-Back - Core and Arm Muscles

These exercises are designed to closely mimic a regular golf swing. The first part of the classic golf swing begins as the body and club are pulled back and up into the pre-swing starting position. Therefore, this first exercise is designed to exercise the muscles involved in pulling the body and golf club back to the starting position. Resistance can be applied at various points along the arc of motion and prevent further movement by gripping the rope harder. This will allow an isometric exercise to be performed, which will build greater strength and power into the overall golf swing movement. To perform this exercise, you will need to use a solid door and doorframe. The door should open inwards so that when resistance is applied against it, the door is pulled closed. A long, sturdy climbing rope is needed, wound into a large ball and then tied and knotted at one end. This will act as a securing mechanism, preventing the rope from slipping under between the door and the floor. It enables you to apply maximum resistance to the rope as you emulate the golf swing motion. To perform the exercise, assume the start of the classic golf swing position, standing close to the door, holding the longer end of the rope. The harder you engage the muscles, the more intense the exercise becomes, so always be sure to exercise at a level of force and intensity that best suits your ability. Perform the exercise in as many positions as you wish. When you perform an isometric exercise, never hold your breath. Always breathe deeply and naturally, which will be about 10 full breaths in and out at a rate of about 1 second per full breath. Perform each exercise for no less than 7 seconds and no longer than 10. NOTE. When applying force to pull on the rope, do so slowly and never suddenly apply maximum force from a cold start. Instead, find each ideal exercise position and gradually increase the applied force until the desired level has been reached. Then, perform the isometric exercise.

Right: The rope knot is now positioned at the bottom of the door on the floor so that the rope can run under the door to exercise with.

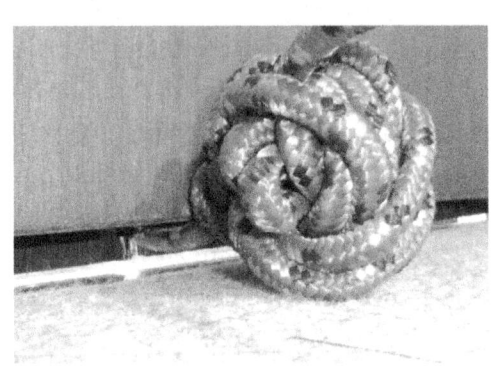

Below: This picture demonstrates how the rope running under the door is used and gripped during the follow-through part of the golf swing.

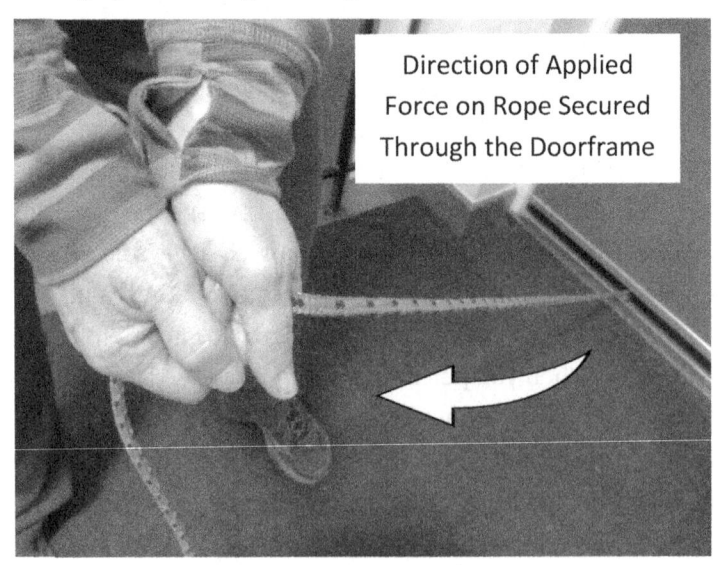

Direction of Applied Force on Rope Secured Through the Doorframe

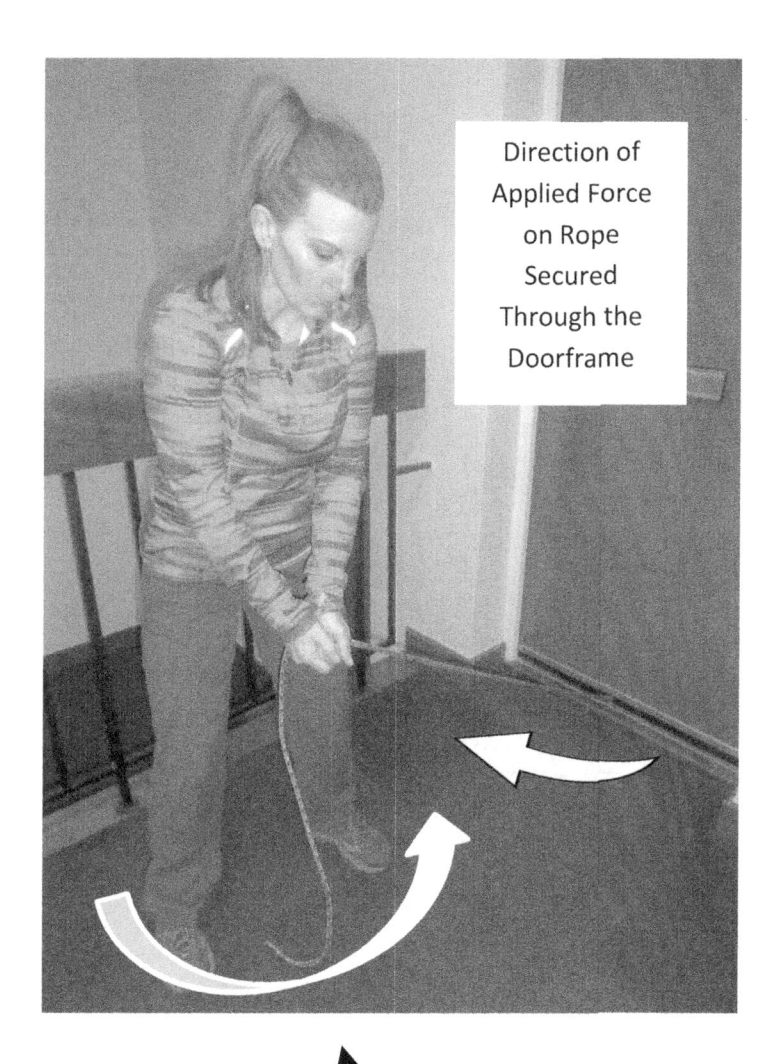

Direction of Applied Force on Rope Secured Through the Doorframe

Direction of Very Slight Body Rotation after Each Exercise to the Next Exercise Position

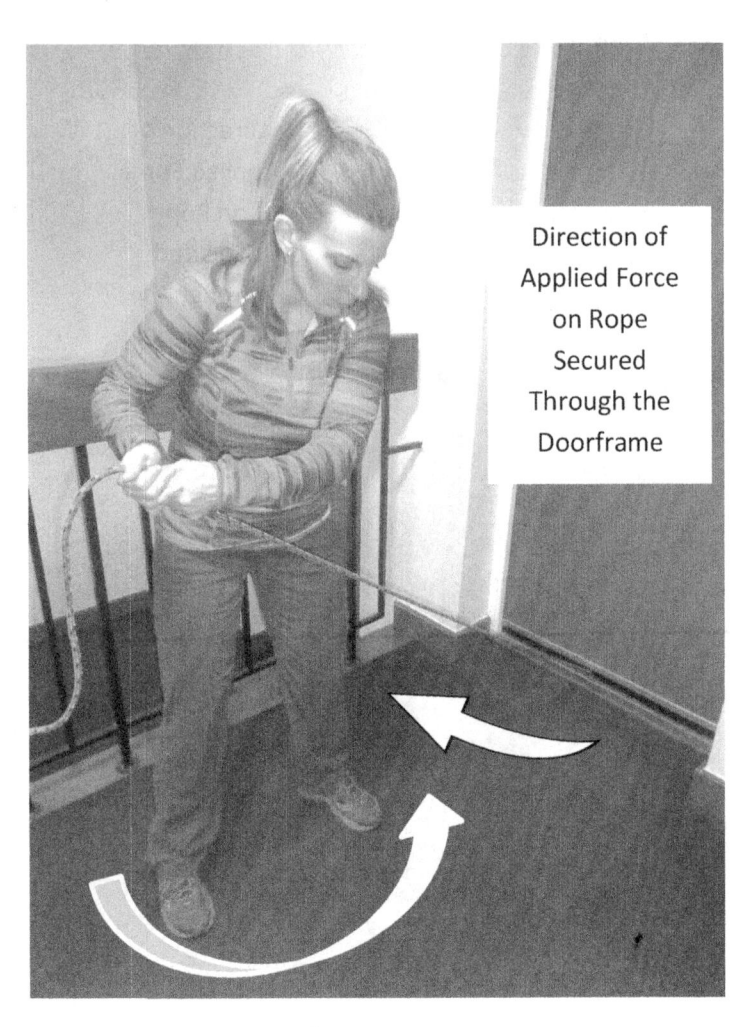

Direction of Applied Force on Rope Secured Through the Doorframe

Direction of Very Slight Body Rotation after Each Exercise to the Next Exercise Position

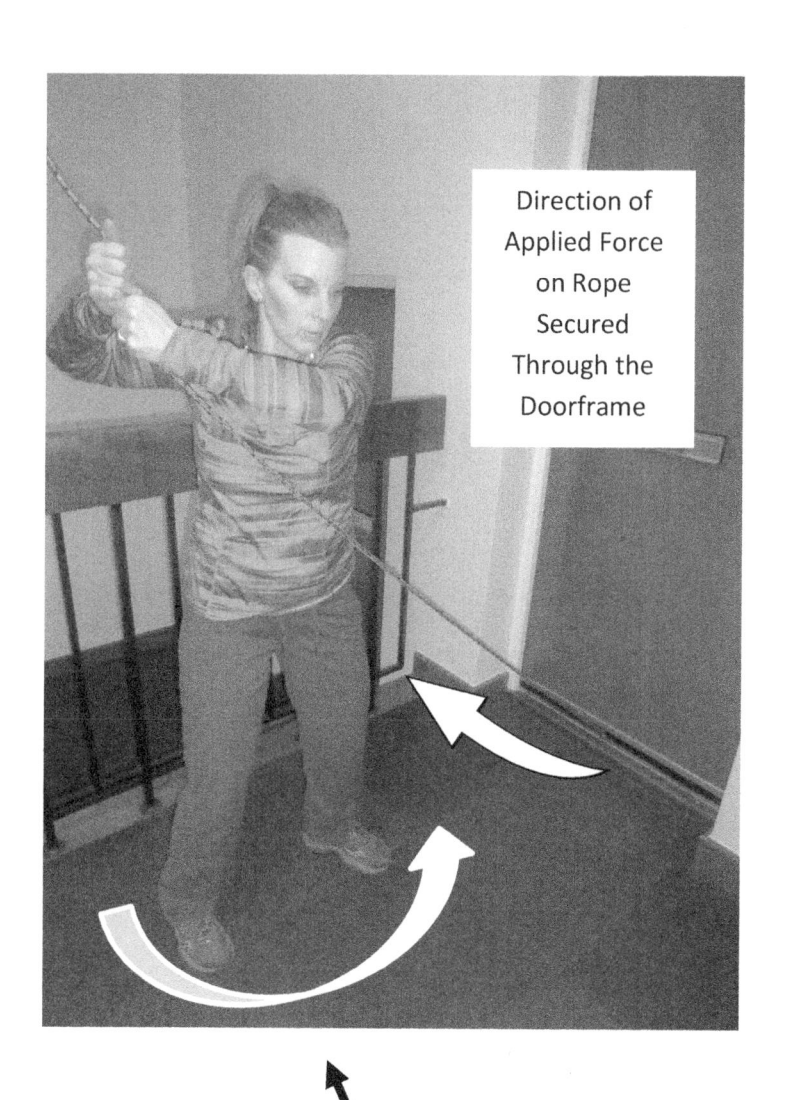

Direction of Applied Force on Rope Secured Through the Doorframe

Direction of Very Slight Body Rotation after Each Exercise to the Next Exercise Position

Golf Swing Door Pull – Core and Arm Muscles

This exercise is designed to closely mimic a regular golf swing. Resistance can be applied at various points along the arc of motion and prevent further movement by gripping the rope harder. This will allow an isometric exercise to be performed, which will build greater strength and power into the overall golf swing movement. To perform this exercise, you will need to use a solid door and doorframe. The door should open inwards so that when resistance is applied against it, the door is pulled closed. A long, sturdy climbing rope is needed, which is wound into a large ball and then tied and knotted at one end. This will act as a securing mechanism, preventing the rope from slipping between the door and the doorframe. It enables you to apply maximum resistance to the rope as you emulate the golf swing motion. To perform the exercise, assume the classic golf swing position, standing close to the door and holding the longer end of the rope. The harder you engage the muscles, the more intense the exercise becomes, so always be sure to exercise at a level of force that best suits your ability. Perform the exercise in as many positions as you wish. When you perform an isometric exercise, never hold your breath. Always breathe deeply and naturally, which will be about 10 full breaths in and out at a rate of about 1 second per full breath. Perform each exercise for no less than 7 seconds and no longer than 10. NOTE. When applying force to pull on the rope, do so slowly and never suddenly apply maximum force from a cold start. Instead, find each ideal exercise position and gradually increase the applied force until the desired level has been reached. Then, perform the isometric exercise.

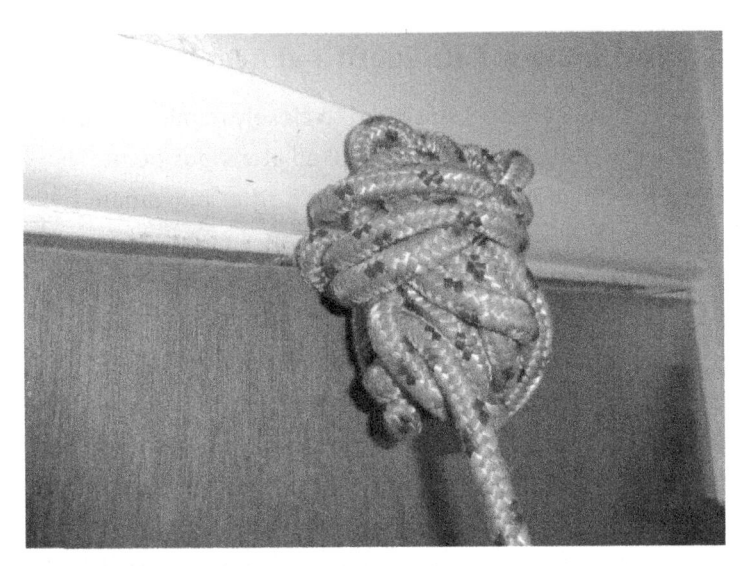

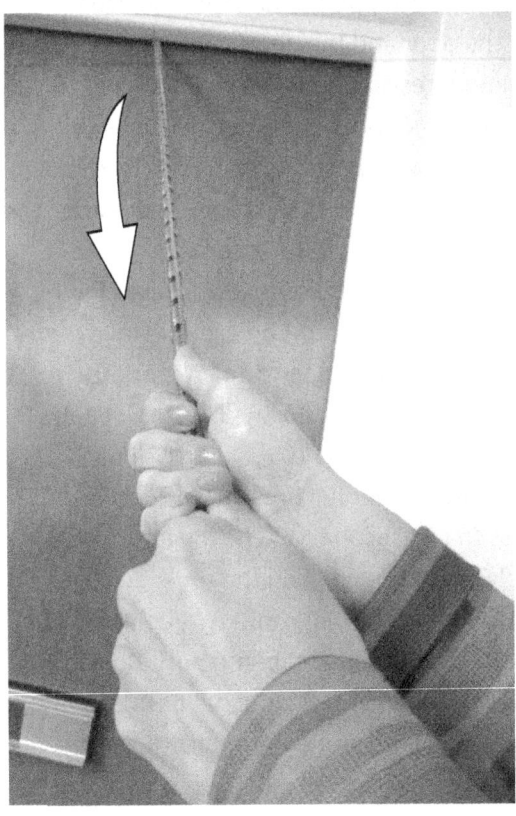

Above: Climbing Rope Ball and Knot Behind the Doorframe

Left: Direction of the Force Applied to Mimicked Golf Swing Action on the Opposite Side of the Door

NOTE. To begin the exercise at the higher end of the golf swing, you must rotate your body slightly away from the door. Similarly, at each point that is chosen to perform an exercise through the range of motion of the swing, the body/foot position will need to rotate slightly accordingly towards the door. This will allow you to emulate the golf swing as closely as possible while at the same time applying the maximum desired force to each isometric exercise.

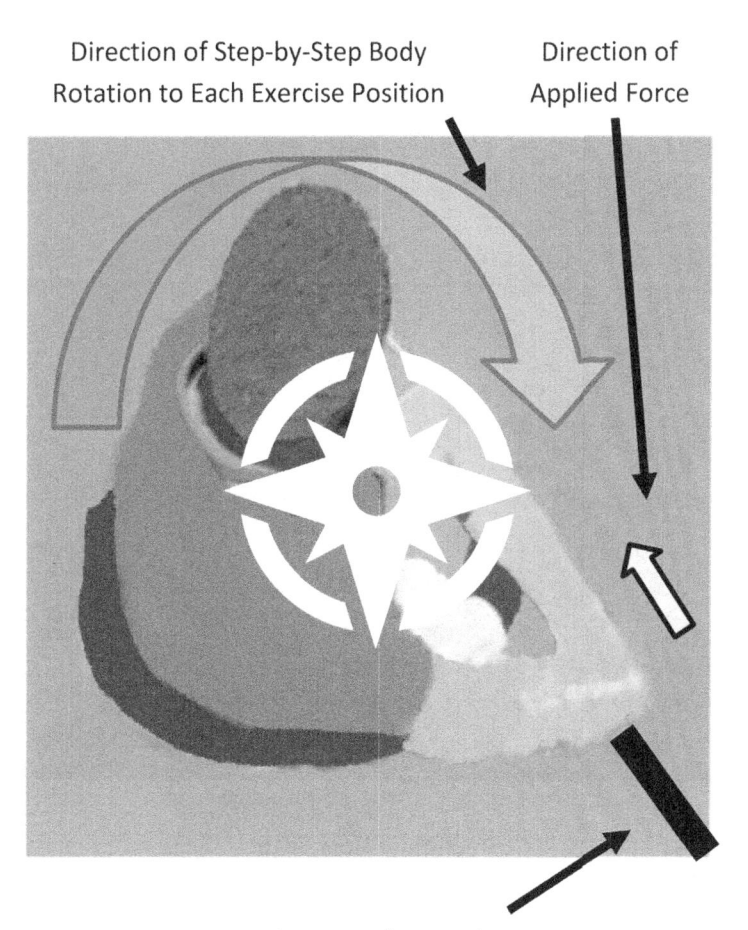

Direction of Step-by-Step Body Rotation to Each Exercise Position

Direction of Applied Force

Rope Leading Back to Doorway Anchor Point

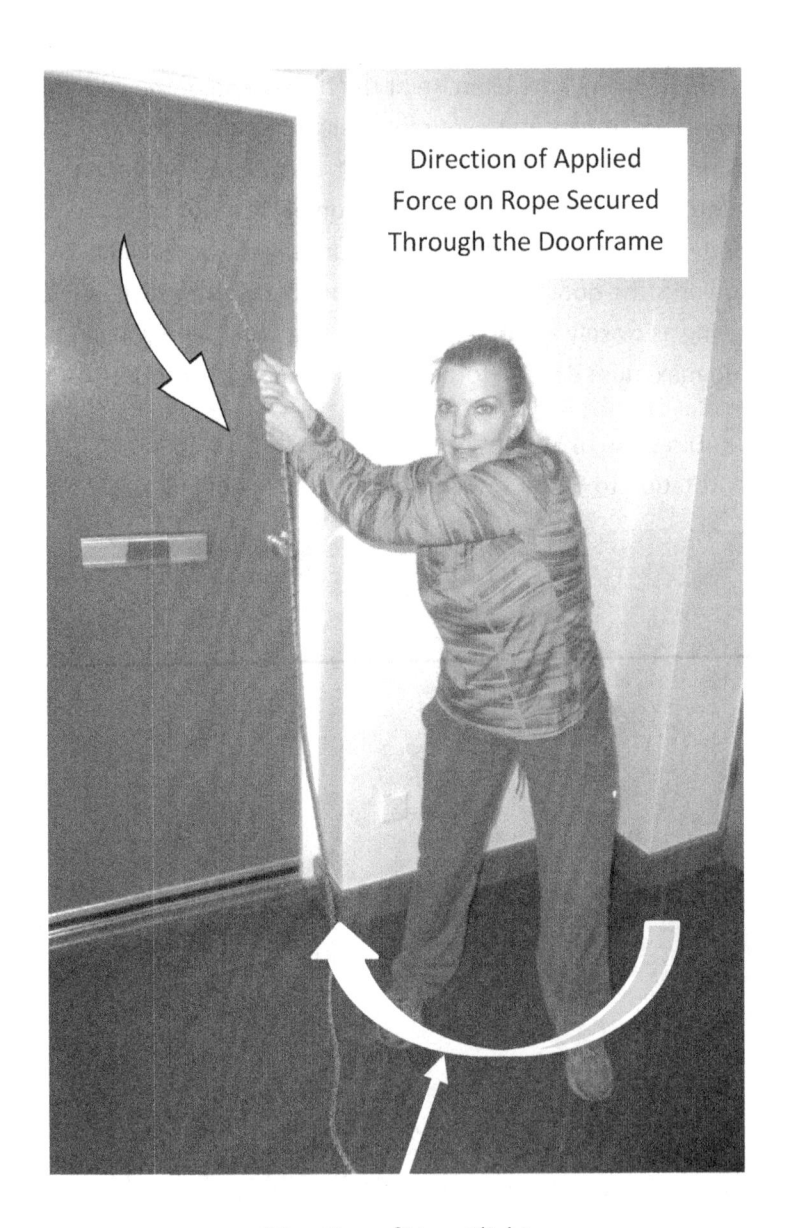

Direction of Applied
Force on Rope Secured
Through the Doorframe

Direction of Very Slight
Body Rotation after
Each Exercise to the
Next Exercise Position

Direction of Applied Force on Rope Secured Through the Doorframe

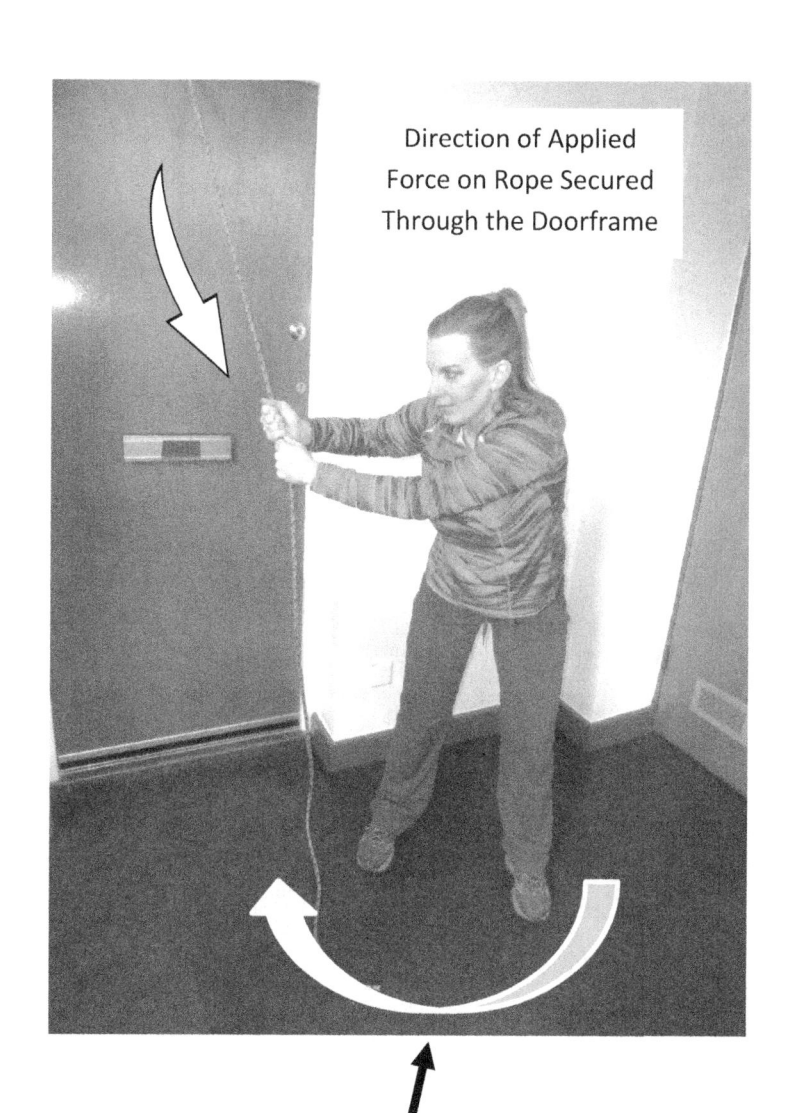

Direction of Very Slight Body Rotation after Each Exercise to the Next Exercise Position

Direction of Applied Force on Rope Secured Through the Doorframe

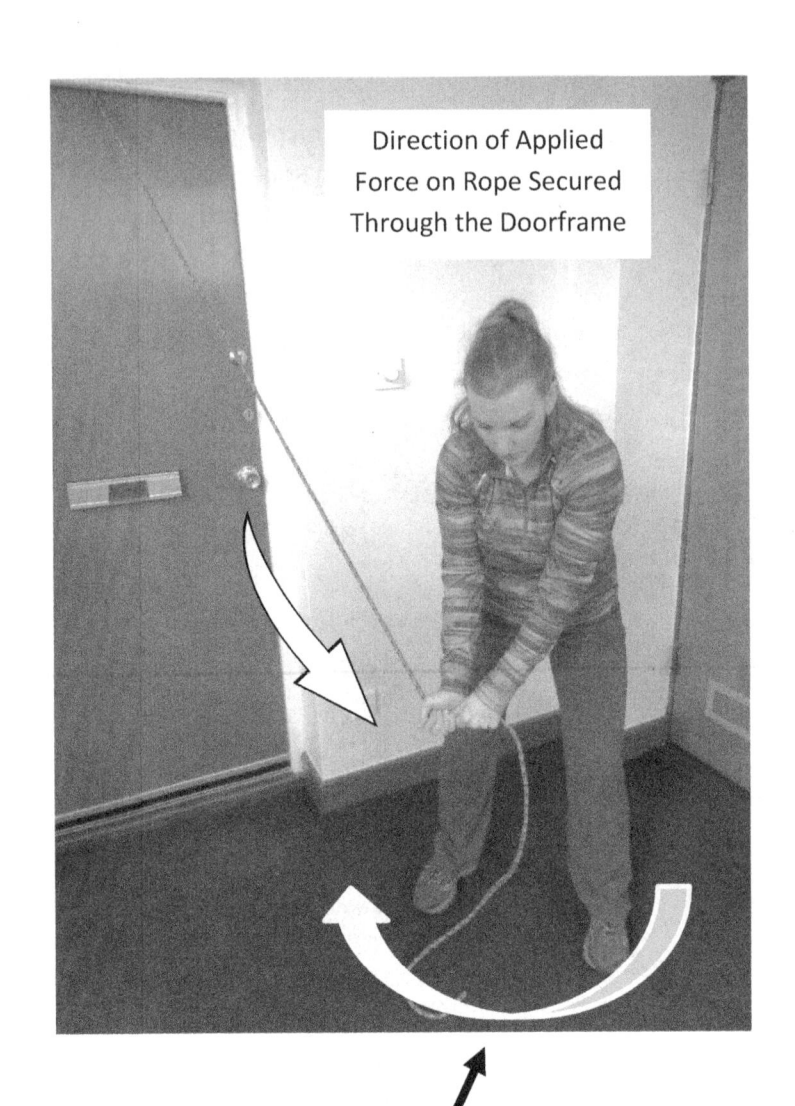

Direction of Very Slight Body Rotation after Each Exercise to the Next Exercise Position

Golf Swing Door Pull – Swing Follow-Through From Centre Point - Core and Arm Muscles

This is the continuation exercise to the previous one, the *Golf Swing Door Pull Core and Arm Muscles*. To perform it, firstly, the climbing rope needs to be repositioned from over the top of a door, to underneath a door. The rope is secured in the same way as in the previous exercise, with the large ball and knot arrangement preventing the rope from being able to be pulled through under the door. The harder you engage the muscles, the more intense the exercise becomes, so always be sure to exercise at a level of force that best suits your ability. When you perform an isometric exercise, never hold your breath. Always breathe deeply and naturally, which will be about 10 full breaths in and out at a rate of about 1 second per full breath. Perform each exercise for no less than 7 seconds and no longer than 10. NOTE. When applying force to pull on the rope, do so slowly and never suddenly apply maximum force from a cold start. Instead, find each ideal exercise position and gradually increase the applied force until the desired level has been reached. Then, perform the isometric exercise.

NOTE. To begin the exercise at the centre point of the golf swing, you will need to position your body in line with the rope under the door. Then, at each chosen point, to perform an exercise through the range of motion of the follow-through of the swing, the body/foot position will need to rotate slightly towards the door. This will allow you to emulate the follow-through of the golf swing as closely as possible while at the same time applying the maximum desired force to each isometric exercise.

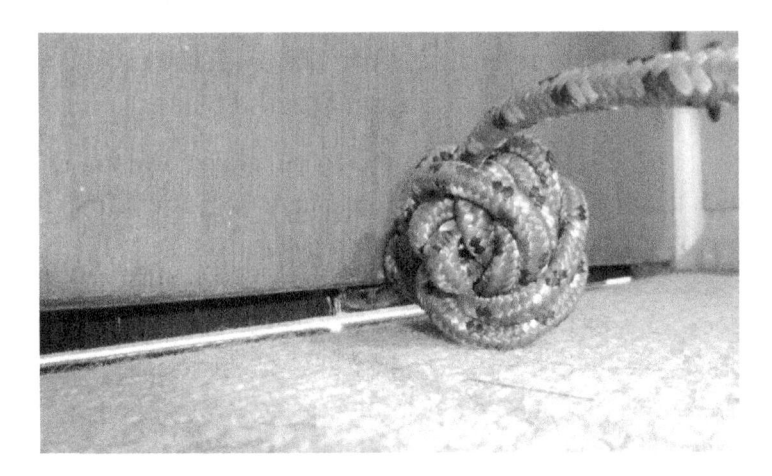

Above: The Rope Knot is Now Positioned at the Bottom of the Door on the Floor so that the Rope can run under the Door to Exercise With.

Below: This Picture is to Demonstrate How the Rope Running Under the Door is Used and Gripped During the Follow-Through Part of the Golf Swing.

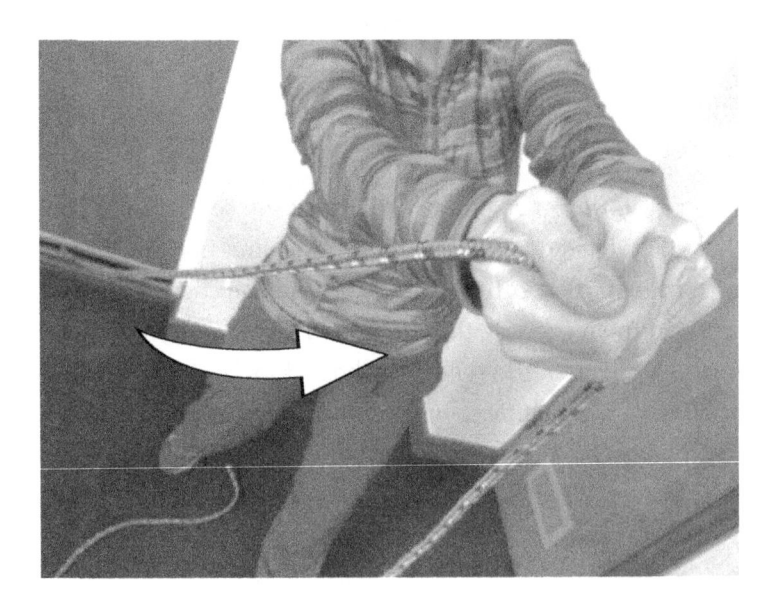

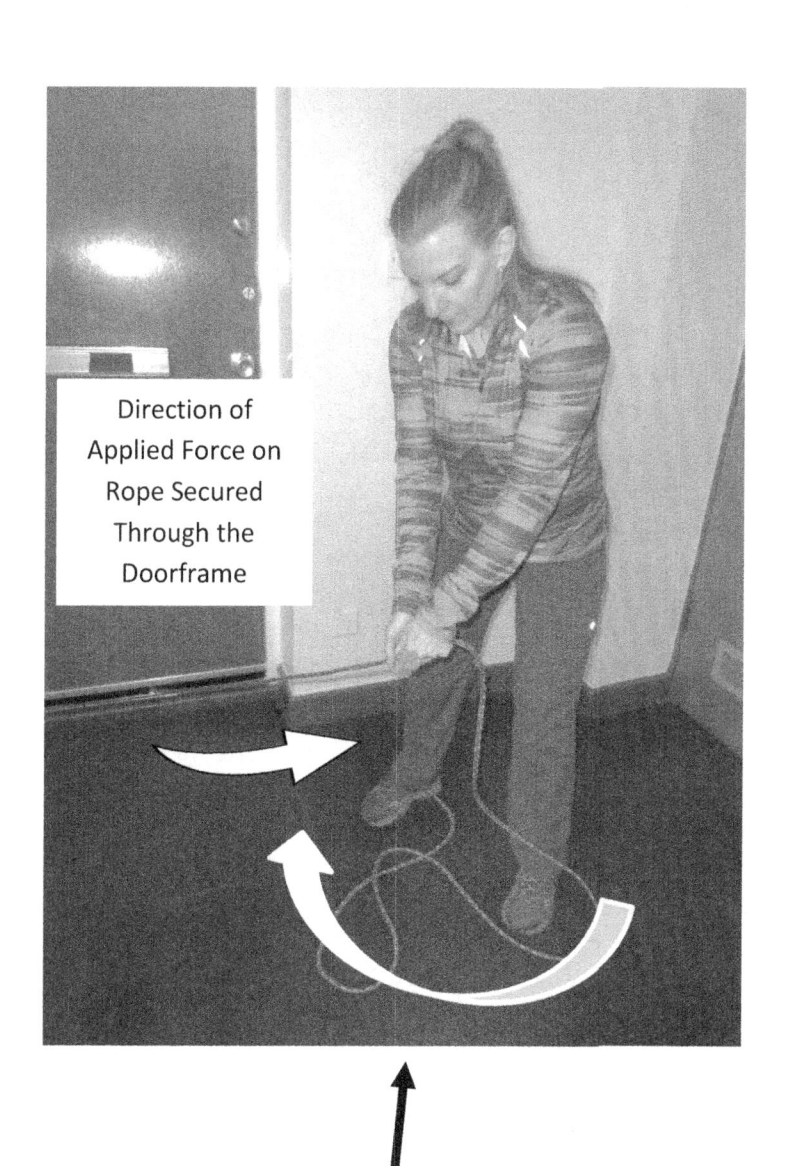

Direction of Applied Force on Rope Secured Through the Doorframe

Direction of Very Slight Body Rotation after Each Exercise to the Next Exercise Position

Direction of Applied Force on Rope Secured Through the Doorframe

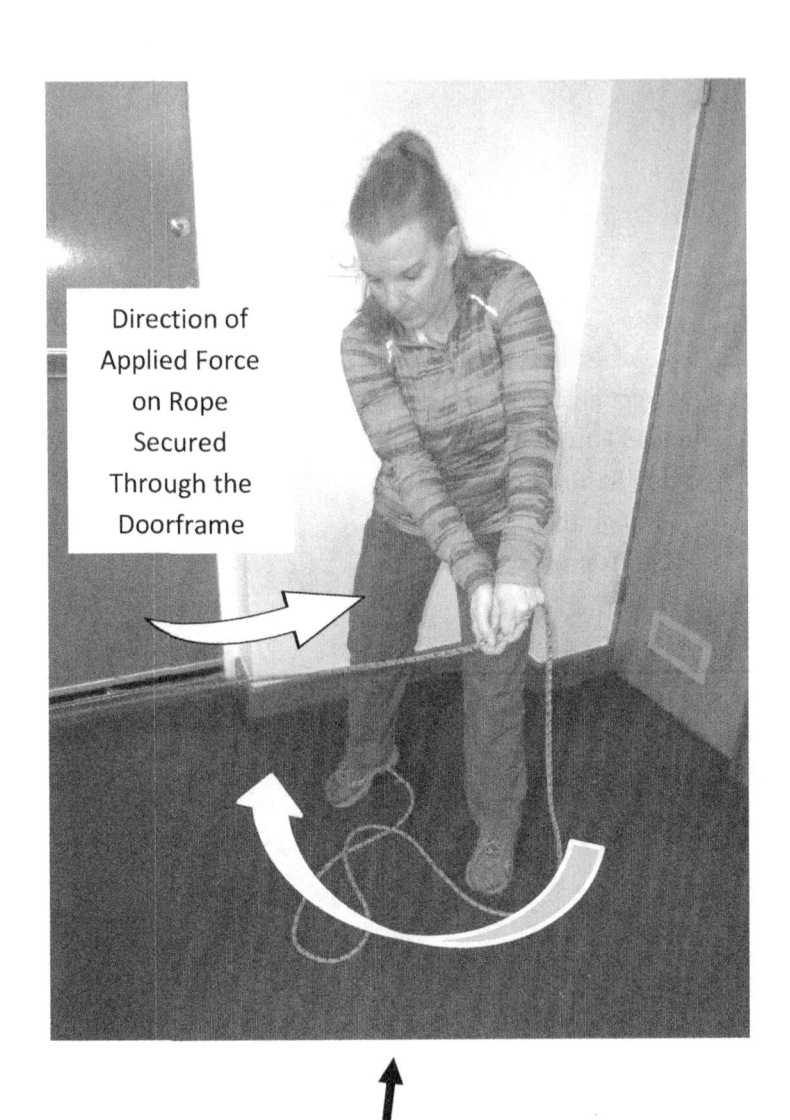

Direction of Very Slight Body Rotation after Each Exercise to the Next Exercise Position

193

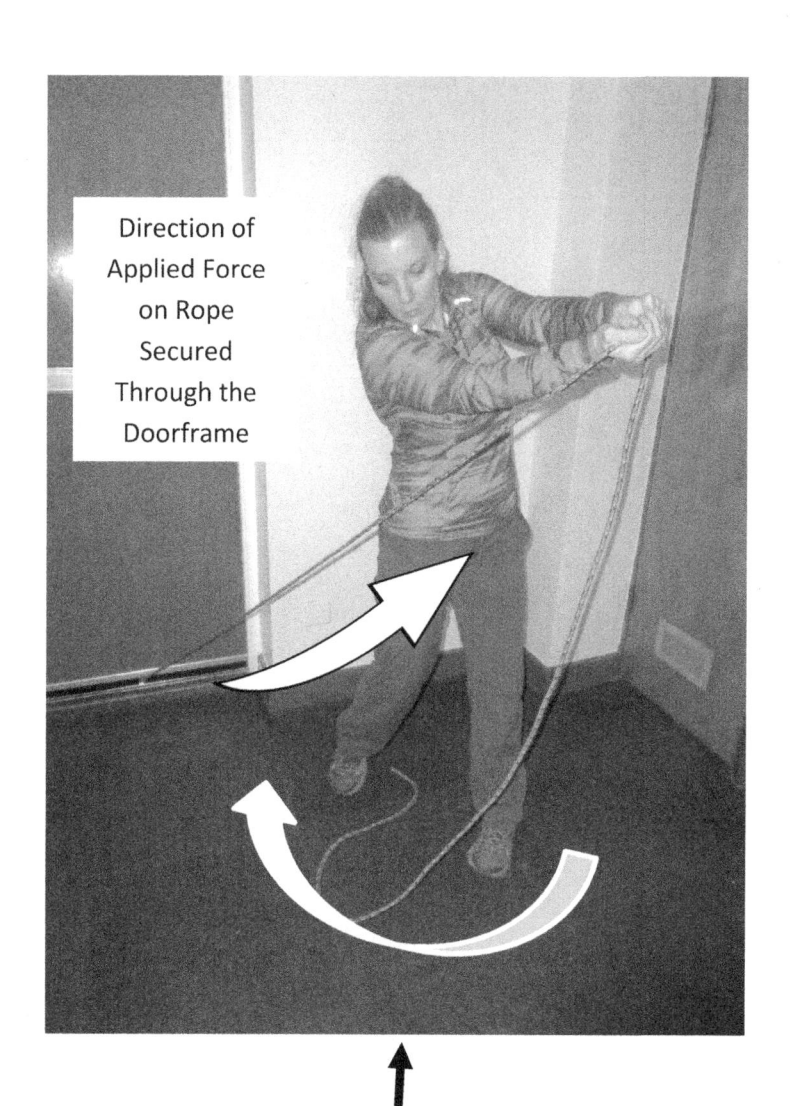

Direction of Applied Force on Rope Secured Through the Doorframe

Direction of Very Slight Body Rotation after Each Exercise to the Next Exercise Position

Chapter 7: Conclusion

Golf is a fun and often challenging game that is also an excellent form of exercise. Furthermore, it can be enjoyed by people of almost all ages and almost all abilities.

It does not matter if you play golf occasionally just for fun; if you are a serious amateur or a full-time professional player, the overall golfing experience can be greatly enhanced by incorporating an isometric exercise routine at some point during the process.

Aside from the proven effectiveness of the exercise system, isometric exercise is quick, easy to perform, and an excellent way to exercise anywhere you choose. One can enjoy a total-body workout routine anywhere with simple yet powerful isometrics. For regular gym users who for years have been caught in the "I can never be too far away from a gym" mental trap, performing isometric exercises is frequently seen as being one of the most freeing experiences imaginable.

When we wrote our book Fitness on the Move™, the isometric exercises we selected to incorporate were the same ones we had been performing ourselves on our worldwide travels over the years. These exercises are similar to many of those in this book, and the technique is always the same.

Isometric exercise has enabled us to enjoy gym-quality total-body workout routines while on the move in some highly unusual places. Once, I performed an isometric exercise routine with the cult moviemaker Cliff Twemlow on the deck of a ship in a storm on the Mediterranean Sea as we travelled from Ibiza to Barcelona. Helen and I have performed total body isometric workout routines on beaches all over the world, from Cornwall to California, on mountainsides, and by lakes and lochs in Cumbria, Scotland, Iceland, and across North America and Canada. We have exercised effectively on long plane journeys without leaving our seats as passengers in cars, buses, and trains. Once, while we were waiting for the rest of our tour party, we even had a "70 Second Difference™" isometric workout 2341 feet underground in the Soudan Mine, on the south shore of Lake Vermilion, in the Vermilion Mountain Range in Minnesota, USA. Thanks to the isometric exercise system, we have been able to exercise anywhere and everywhere we want to.

One of the best things about it all has been that to perform a total-body workout routine, we typically needed no equipment or only the bare minimum that could easily fit into our pockets. After reading this book, you now know that you can perform a highly effective isometric exercise routine with nothing except your bare hands.

However, by using what we call IIEDs, or Improvised Isometric Exercise Devices, such as a golf club, climbing rope, martial arts or regular belts, golf clubs, walking poles, or the amazing Iso-Bow™, you can carry a powerful portable gymnasium with you wherever you go.

Now that you know how the isometric exercise system works, you also know how all the aforementioned IIEDs can be used effectively to deliver a powerful and efficient workout wherever you choose to perform one.

Isometric exercise should not be performed only outdoors during golfing practice or a friendly game.

Incorporating a regular isometric exercise routine into your daily schedule at home or work will deliver amazing benefits for your overall strength, fitness, and body shape.

Your newfound fitness and strength will bring many additional benefits. It will make general daily tasks easier to perform, and for many, it will mean that they will perform better at their chosen sports or physical pastimes.

Crucially, for some, regular isometric exercise will greatly improve their overall mobility and performance when it comes to climbing stairs and standing up from a chair unaided. Whatever one does in life that is physical, being stronger and fitter always makes it easier and more fun. Let isometric exercise be your key to unleashing your full potential regardless of your current age or physical ability.

Many serious golfers and professional golf coaches are now recognising the value and effectiveness of isometric exercise for themselves and their clients. As such, they are choosing to become accredited isometric exercise instructors through TWiEA, The World Isometric Exercise Association. This enables them to deliver safe, effective, and enhanced exercise coaching anywhere they choose during practice sessions or breaks during a friendly game. We wish you every success in life and sincerely thank you for taking the time to read this book and to hopefully perform isometric exercises regularly. For more information, visit www.TWiEA.com

www.HelenRenee.com – www.BrianSterlingVete.com

What is TWiEA™?

TWiEA™ is the acronym for The World Isometric Exercise Association, the global governing body for all types of isometric exercise. TWiEA™'s mission is to help set and maintain standards of excellence in teaching and promoting all types of isometric exercise.

TWiEA™'s mission is to ensure that scientifically proven time-efficient isometric exercise techniques are taught to clients as part of an integrated overall approach to the total-body exercise solutions provided by fitness professionals. This creates a much higher probability that busy clients often face real-life time crunches and can still maintain a regular, highly effective exercise program.

The fact is that isometric exercise is every bit as effective, and frequently more effective, at building muscle and strength as other more traditional forms of resistance training. It is also a time-saving and money-saving exercise solution that almost anyone can perform, even without equipment.

www.HelenRenee.com – www.BrianSterlingVete.com

Other books by Brian Sterling-Vete and Helen Renée Wuorio

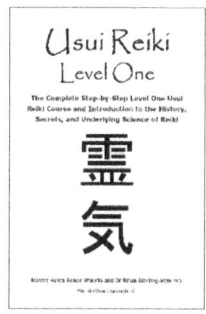

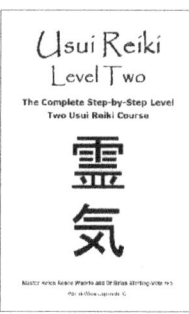

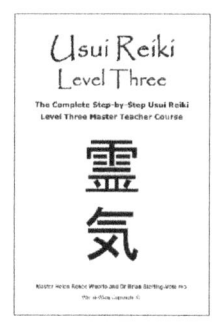

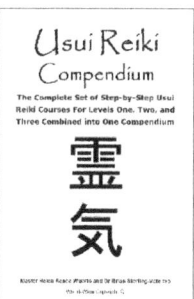

Usui Reiki Level One

A comprehensive introduction to Reiki, its history, and the science. This course is written in an easy-to-follow step-by-step way, so you know exactly what to do and when to do it. This and other books in the series also serve as course manuals for our Reiki students.

Usui Reiki Level Two

The Reiki Level Two course is the next step in your Reiki journey teaching the Power Symbols and how to use them. It is laid out in an easy-to-understand step-by-step way so you will know exactly what to do and when to do it.

Usui Reiki Level Three

The Level Three Master Teacher course is the final step after Level Two. It is laid out logically in an easy-to-understand step-by-step way so you will know exactly what to do and when to do it.

Usui Reiki Compendium – Levels 1 & 2

The Reiki Compendium is a complete and unabridged book of our Usui Reiki Level One and Two courses. It's ideal for those wishing to progress right through both levels. This and other books in the series also serve as course manuals for our online or in-person Reiki Students.

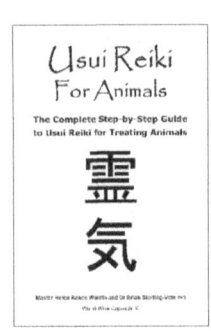

Usui Reiki for Treating Animals

This is ideal for practitioners at any level who want to learn techniques for treating animals safely and effectively. It also covers the differences in animal chakras and energy centres and those unique to certain animals.

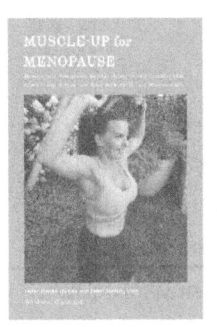

Muscle-up For Menopause

Approved by TWiEA – The World Isometric Exercise Association. Menopause cannot be avoided, so take control of every element possible. Brief yet intense exercise sessions that place the minimum demand on your ability to recover, combined with a high-protein plant-based diet, can make all the difference between making life easier or harder during menopause. This course can be performed with or without equipment.

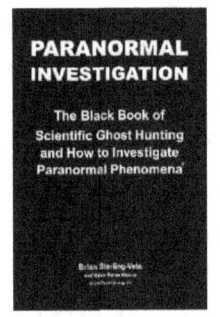

Paranormal Investigation - The Black Book of Scientific Ghost Hunting and How to Investigate Paranormal Phenomena™

This best-selling book is ideal for beginners and advanced investigators who want to apply a more scientific approach. It contains a special scientific critical path graphic page to work from and a step-by-step guide to a complete paranormal investigation. It also tells you how to protect yourself from malevolent paranormal entities.

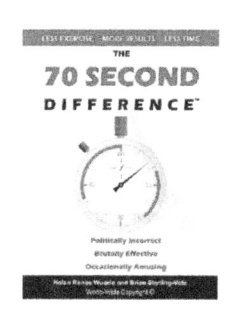

The 70 Second Difference™ - The Politically Incorrect, Occasionally Amusing, and Brutally Effective Guide to Strength, Fitness and Better Health

Approved by TWiEA – The World Isometric Exercise Association.

This is a science-based, no-nonsense guide about the most efficient ways to exercise, build muscle and strength, and how lifestyle and dietary choices affect you. Just 70 seconds a day of focused science-based exercise can give you a total-body workout.

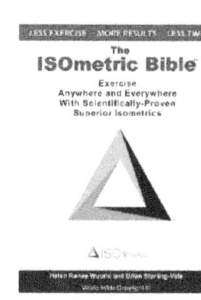

The ISOmetric Bible™ - Exercise Anywhere with Scientifically Proven Isometrics

Approved by TWiEA – The World Isometric Exercise Association.

A complete, practical, scientific, and user-friendly benchmark book about scientifically proven isometric exercise. No special equipment is needed for a total-body workout.

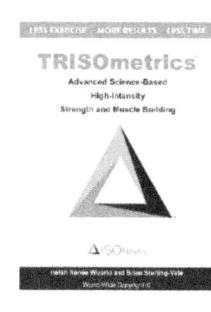

TRISOmetrics™ - Advanced Science-Based High-Intensity Strength and Muscle Building

Approved by TWiEA – The World Isometric Exercise Association.

An advanced, science-based, high-intensity exercise system combines 3 scientifically proven techniques into a powerful new system. It can be performed with or without equipment when travelling or as part of a gym-based exercise routine.

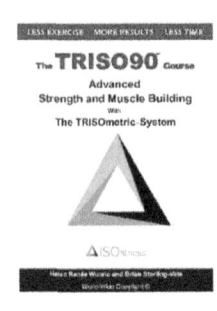

The TRISO90™ Course – Advanced Strength and Muscle Building with The TRISOmetrics™ System

Approved by TWiEA – The World Isometric Exercise Association.

A 90-day/12-week step-by-step highly advanced bodybuilding/shaping and strength-training exercise course. It combines three proven science-based principles. It can be performed with or without equipment or as part of a gym-based exercise routine.

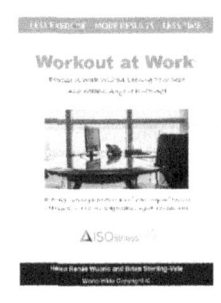

Workout at Work™ - Exercise at Work Without Anyone Even Knowing What You're Doing!

Approved by TWiEA – The World Isometric Exercise Association.

Time is the #1 reason why people do not exercise. The average person spends over 10 years of their life at a desk! You can exercise effectively without leaving your desk with scientifically proven isometric exercise.

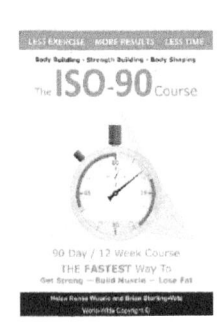

The ISO90™ Course – The 12-Week/90-Day Shape-up and Get Strong Course

Approved by TWiEA – The World Isometric Exercise Association.

This complete, step-by-step 90-day/12-week isometric body shaping, bodybuilding, and strength-building course is ideal for beginners and advanced trainers.

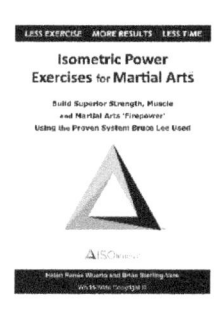

Isometric Power Exercises for Martial Arts™ - Build Superior Strength, Muscle and Martial Arts 'Firepower' Using the Proven System Bruce Lee Used

Approved by TWiEA – The World Isometric Exercise Association.

This book is a valuable resource for practical isometric exercises to build serious strength, muscle, and martial arts firepower.

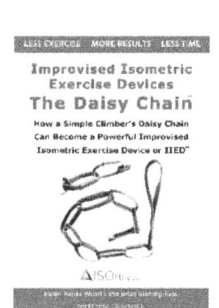

Improvised Isometric Exercise Devices - The Daisy Chain - How a Simple Climber's Daisy Chain Can Become a Powerful Improvised Isometric Exercise Device or IIED

Approved by TWiEA – The World Isometric Exercise Association.

Improvised Isometric Exercise Devices, or IIEDs, come in all shapes and sizes and are only limited by your imagination. This is a valuable resource listing practical exercises that can be performed and how to extend the daisy chain safely.

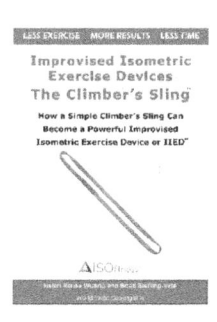

The Climber's Sling - How a Simple Climber's Sling Can Become a Powerful Improvised Isometric Device or IIED

Approved by TWiEA – The World Isometric Exercise Association.

IIEDs come in all shapes and sizes and are only limited by your imagination. This is a valuable resource listing practical isometric exercises that can be performed as well as how to extend the climber's sling safely.

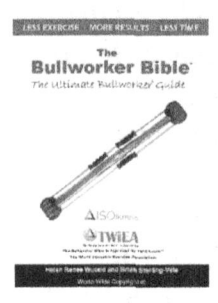

The Bullworker Bible™ The Ultimate Science-Based Guide to The Classic Personal Multi-Gym
Approved by TWiEA – The World Isometric Exercise Association. and the makers of The Bullworker. The original and best guide for all Bullworker® users and the companion book to The Bullworker 90™ Course. It is complete, science-based, and user-friendly, showing how the device should be used to deliver maximum results. Also essential for the Steel Bow®.

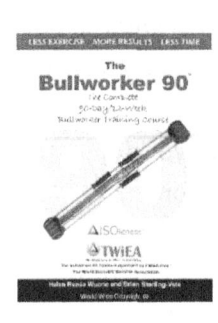

The Bullworker 90™ Course – The Ultimate Science-Based 12-Week/90-Day Get Strong and Grow Muscle Course Using the Classic Personal Multi-Gym
Approved by TWiEA – The World Isometric Exercise Association. and the makers of The Bullworker. A 90-day/12-week step-by-step course for all Bullworker® users and is the companion book to The Bullworker Bible™. Each week has a detailed note section, so you know exactly what to do and when to do it.

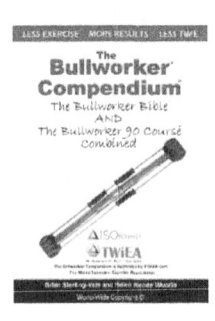

The Bullworker Compendium™ - The Bullworker Bible™ and The Bullworker90™ Course Combined
Approved by TWiEA – The World Isometric Exercise Association. and the makers of The Bullworker. The Bullworker Compendium™ combines both The Bullworker Bible™ and The Bullworker 90™ Course in a single huge book.

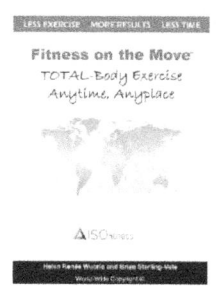

Fitness on the Move™ - Enjoy Gym-Quality Workout Sessions ANYWHERE!
Approved by TWiEA – The World Isometric Exercise Association. This book lists practical exercises that can be performed while travelling almost anywhere and in any vehicle. If there is enough space to sit down and/or stand upright, you can perform a total-body workout!

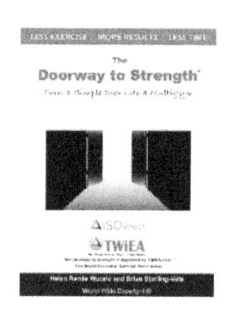

The Doorway to Strength™ - Turn a Door into a Strength-Building Multigym
Approved by TWiEA – The World Isometric Exercise Association. It shows how a simple door, doorway, and frame can be used to create a multi-gym of exercises using the amazing Iso-Bow®. Required: 2 x Iso-Bows®, a solid door and frame, and a door wedge/stop.

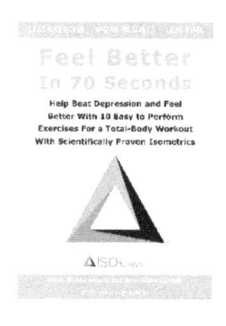

Feel Better In 70 Seconds™
Approved by TWiEA – The World Isometric Exercise Association. Studies indicate that exercising, even briefly, combats depression without needing much money, time, or space. Just 70 seconds of continuous movement enables a 10-exercise, full-body workout through the efficient isometric exercise system. Required: 2 x Iso-Bows®

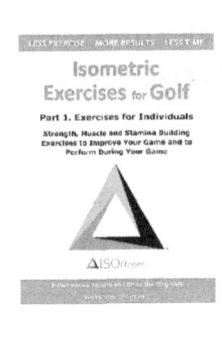

Isometric Exercises for Golf™ Part 1. Exercises for Individuals. Approved by TWiEA – The World Isometric Exercise Association. Isometric exercises, ideal for game or practice, can transform a round of golf into a full-body workout when performed at each of the 18 holes using a golf club as an improvised exercise device. Part 1 serves as a guide, offering tailored exercises to enhance swing power for those with specific needs.

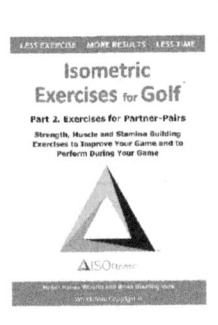

Isometric Exercises for Golf™ Part 2. Partner-Pairs

Approved by TWiEA – The World Isometric Exercise Association. The companion to Book 1 focuses on exercises best performed in partnered pairs during a break, a game, or practice sessions.

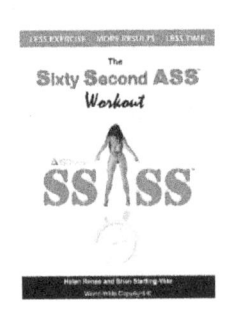

The Sixty Second ASS Workout™ - The Ultimate 60-Second Workout to Shape, Tone, Lift, and Give You the Backside You've Always Wanted

Approved by TWiEA – The World Isometric Exercise Association. The fastest and most effective "ass" workout ever devised. Scientifically proven exercises deliver a no-nonsense, time-efficient workout.

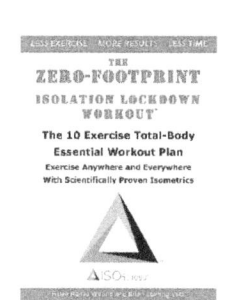

The Zero-Footprint Isolation Lockdown Workout - The 10 Exercise Total-Body Essential Workout - Approved by TWiEA – The World Isometric Exercise Association. 10 essential total-body exercises can be performed anywhere; if you can stand and sit, you can perform a powerful workout routine in as little as 70 seconds a day! NOTE: This is a variation of The 70 Second Difference™ workout.

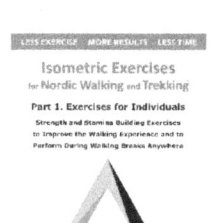

Isometric Exercises for Nordic Walking and Trekking™ - Part 1. Exercises for Individuals. Approved by TWiEA – The World Isometric Exercise Association. Perform gym-quality total-body isometric exercise routines during walk breaks almost anywhere using walking/trekking poles as an IIED or Improvised Isometric Exercise Device. Book 1. is a resource guide of exercises performed by individuals.

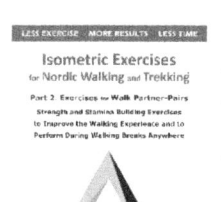

Isometric Exercises for Nordic Walking and Trekking™ - Part 2. Exercises for Walk Partner-Pairs
Approved by TWiEA – The World Isometric Exercise Association.
This is the companion to Book 1 and is focused on exercises that are best performed as a partner-pair, with a friend.

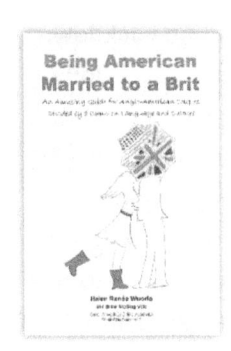

Being American Married to a Brit™ - An Amusing Guide for Anglo-American Couples Divided by a Common Language and Culture

A quirky, eye-opening, and fun-filled roller-coaster ride about how even the most basic everyday transatlantic conversations can bring laughter. It is dedicated to all transatlantic couples who are divided and confused by their common language.

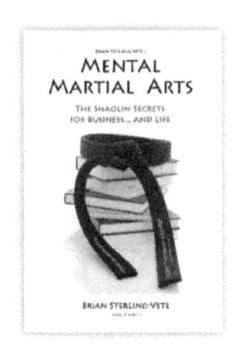

Mental Martial Arts™ - intellectual Life and Business Combat Skills

A system of intellectual language and life-combat skills using the tactics and principles of physical martial arts. How to verbally and intellectually guide, channel, and redirect the energy of powerful people and large organisations to achieve the outcomes that you desire.

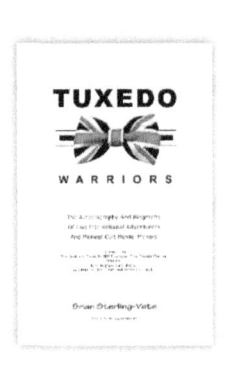

Tuxedo Warriors™

The companion book to The Tuxedo Warrior and the movie is the biography and autobiography of the iconic cult author, composer, and moviemaker Cliff Twemlow. It continues the story from where Cliff's book finishes and is the most complete biography of Cliff Twemlow ever written, covering the late 1970s to his death. It is also the autobiography of Brian Sterling-Vete.

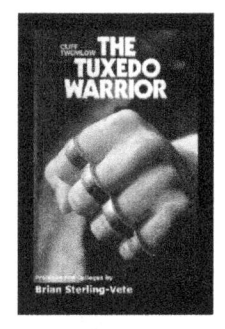

The Tuxedo Warrior™ by Cliff Twemlow – Prologue and epilogue by Brian Sterling-Vete. A Doorman navigates respect with diplomacy or force, managing nightlife's challenges. "The Tuxedo Warrior" reveals this balancing act, depicting peaceful resolutions or violent clashes, providing a raw glimpse into the vibrant yet perilous world of nighttime order-keeping.

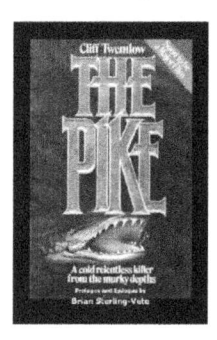

The Pike™ by Cliff Twemlow – Prologue and epilogue by Brian Sterling-Vete. A monstrous pike turns Lake Windermere into a nightmare, attacking people and boats and creating panic among both experts and holidaymakers. Amidst the growing fear, some traders exploit the chaos, hindering the creature's capture to benefit from the intrigued onlookers as the terror escalates.

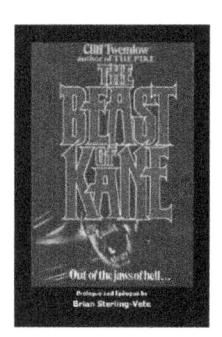

The Beast of Kane™ by Cliff Twemlow – Prologue and epilogue by Brian Sterling-Vete. Unaware, the Gordon Family invites darkness by adopting a stray Elkhound, igniting unheeded prophecies of evil. Kane faces a spree of supernatural terror, from animal attacks to a brutal murder, as a chilling winter amplifies the fear gripping the town.

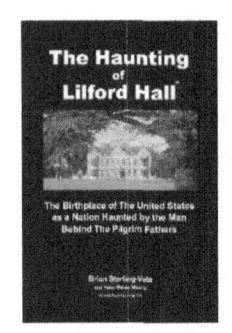

The Haunting of Lilford Hall™ - The Birthplace of the United States as a Nation Haunted by the Man Behind The Pilgrim Fathers. This is one of the most baffling cases ever recorded of paranormal activity experienced by multiple people between 2012 and 2013. Robert Browne is the man responsible for getting the Pilgrim Fathers to sail on The Mayflower in 1620, and it is believed that his ghost still haunts Lilford Hall.

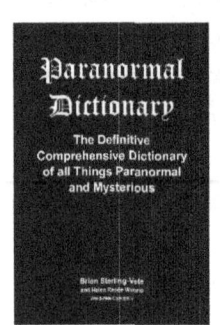

Paranormal Dictionary
A complete and comprehensive guide to all of the most common paranormal terminology, entities, and equipment used during investigations, plus a few enduring mysteries for good measure. It is ideal for both new and experienced investigators.

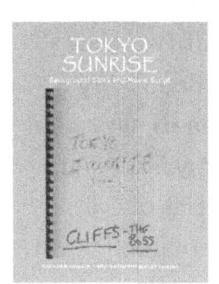

Tokyo Sunrise Background and Script
This was one of Cliff Twemlow's famous films that was never completed, even after extensive filming by Robert Foster, the great cinematographer, to produce a promo video to try to sell the movie to investors. This tells the background story and the Richard Gere connection.

Hair Transplantation and Restoration

This is the essential complete guide to hair loss, growth, and all hair transplantation and restoration forms. It is a collaboration between Brian Sterling-Vete and Malcolm Mendelsohn, the world's #1 independent expert with almost 50 years of experience.

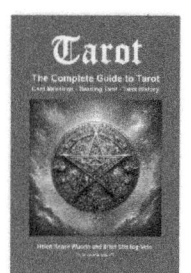

Tarot – The Complete Guide

The ultimate tarot guidebook covers the rich history, diverse styles of cards, and their meanings. Learn the art of tarot reading with comprehensive insights and techniques in one authoritative source. Unlock your tarot journey today.

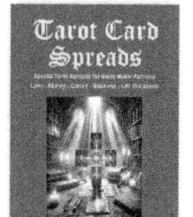

Tarot Card Spreads

The definitive tarot card spread guidebook offers an array of spreads for every major purpose, including love, money, career, business, and crucial life decisions. It contains detailed diagrams, descriptions, and their applications. Elevate your tarot practice with this indispensable resource.

www.HelenRenee.com – www.BrianSterlingVete.com

Made in the USA
Coppell, TX
14 January 2025